the Unofficial Guide™ to Cosmetic Surgery

E. Bingo Wyer

Macmillan • USA

Macmillan General Reference
A Simon & Schuster Macmillan Company
1633 Broadway
New York, New York 10019-6785

ISBN: 0-02-862522-6

Manufactured in the United States of America

10 9 8 7 6 5 4 3 2 1

First edition

For Neal,
plucky researcher, adorable father

Acknowledgments

Without the generous help of many doctors, this book would be a pamphlet. The indefatigable, generous, and enormously skilled Dr. Gregory LaTrenta exceeded all expectations. I'm ever grateful. Thanks to doctors Sherrell J. Aston, Stephen P. Grifka, Sue Ellen Cox, Robert N. Cooper, Z. Paul Lorenc, Gerald Imber, Douglas D. Dedo, Joshua L. Fox, Zein E. Obagi, and so many others.

I'm grateful to Nohmie B. Myers and Maureen and Ed Rover for their great charm and endless support. My Malibu alter ego, Kathleen Wyer, introduced me to Macmillan and offered great optimism in the face of El Niño. Thank you. Bruce and Minette Nelson, Reed and Lily, too, cheered me in more ways than they might imagine; I become lost without you. Sylvia Burt, tireless advisor and friend: Thank you.

Creative fireball Helene Schoenfeld (as well as Howard and Marcia), literary agent Stedman Mays, and the tireless Renee Lord assured me impossible hurdles are always a breeze. I have scanned you all into my heart.

Old friends never die; they don't even get wrinkles. The endless help of Anne Kitchens, Timothy Callaghan, Peter Essex, Helen Ginns, Joe Godfrey, Jo Bishop, Lin Braun, Dr. Leslie Gold, Lynn Wilde, Frank X. Fallon, Elizabeth Ahrens, and Victoria Geibel buoy me still.

The cosmetic surgery field is continually enhanced by the best and the brightest, namely Wendy Lewis, Kate Altork, Barbara Rhea, Peggy Broderick, and Debbie Then.

Macmillan is especially fortunate, as am I, to have Jennifer Farthing, Jennifer Perillo, and Bob Shuman; they never let a good night's rest interfere with progress. Finally, but really primarily, there's Lynn Northrup. Eventually she will explain how she learned at the knee of Max Perkins, despite her youth. Right now she's too busy cleaning up my trail. Thank you very much.

Contents

The *Unofficial Guide* Reader's Bill of Rights

We Give You More Than the Official Line

Welcome to the *Unofficial Guide* series of Lifestyles titles—books that deliver critical, unbiased information that other books can't or won't reveal—*the inside scoop*. Our goal is to provide you with the *most accessible, useful* information and advice possible. The recommendations we offer in these pages are not influenced by the corporate line of any organization or industry; we give you the hard facts, whether those institutions like them or not. If something is ill-advised or will cause a loss of time and/or money, we'll give you ample warning. And if it is a worthwhile option, we'll let you know that, too.

Armed and Ready

Our hand-picked authors confidently and critically report on a wide range of topics that matter to smart readers like you. Our authors are passionate about their subjects, but have distanced themselves enough from them to help you be armed and protected, and help you make educated decisions as you go through your process. It is our intent that, from having read this book, you will avoid the pitfalls everyone else falls into and get it right the first time.

Don't be fooled by cheap imitations; this is the genuine article *Unofficial Guide* series from Macmillan Publishing. You may be familiar with our proven track record of the travel *Unofficial Guides,* which have more than three million copies in print. Each year thousands of travelers—new and old—are armed with a brand new, fully updated edition of the flagship *Unofficial Guide to Walt Disney World,* by Bob Sehlinger. It is our intention here to provide you with the same level of objective authority that Mr. Sehlinger does in his brainchild.

The Unofficial Panel of Experts

Every work in the Lifestyle *Unofficial Guides* is intensively inspected by a team of three top professionals in their fields. These experts review the manuscript for factual accuracy, comprehensiveness, and an insider's determination as to whether the manuscript fulfills the credo in this Reader's Bill of Rights. In other words, our Panel ensures that you are, in fact, getting "the inside scoop."

Our Pledge

The authors, the editorial staff, and the Unofficial Panel of Experts assembled for *Unofficial Guides* are determined to lay out the most valuable alternatives available for our readers. This dictum means that our writers must be explicit, prescriptive, and above all, direct. We strive to be thorough and complete, but our goal is not necessarily to have the "most" or "all" of the information on a topic; this is not, after all, an encyclopedia. Our objective is to help you narrow down your options to the best of what is available, unbiased by affiliation with any industry or organization.

In each *Unofficial Guide* we give you:

- Comprehensive coverage of necessary and vital information

- Authoritative, rigidly fact-checked data

- The most up-to-date insights into trends

- Savvy, sophisticated writing that's also readable

- Sensible, applicable facts and secrets that only an insider knows

Special Features

Every book in our series offers the following six special sidebars in the margins that were devised to help you get things done cheaply, efficiently, and smartly.

1. "Timesaver"—tips and shortcuts that save you time.

2. "Moneysaver"—tips and shortcuts that save you money.

3. "Watch Out!"—more serious cautions and warnings.

4. "Bright Idea"—general tips and shortcuts to help you find an easier or smarter way to do something.

5. "Quote"—statements from real people that are intended to be prescriptive and valuable to you.

6. "Unofficially..."—an insider's fact or anecdote.

We also recognize your need to have quick information at your fingertips, and have thus provided the following comprehensive sections at the back of the book:

1. **Glossary:** Definitions of complicated terminology and jargon.

2. **Resource Guide:** Lists of relevant agencies, associations, institutions, web sites, etc.

3. **Recommended Reading List:** Suggested titles that can help you get more in-depth information on related topics.

4. **Important Documents:** "Official" pieces of information you need to refer to, such as government forms.

5. **Important Statistics:** Facts and numbers presented at-a-glance for easy reference.

6. **Index.**

Letters, Comments, and Questions from Readers

We strive to continually improve the *Unofficial* series, and input from our readers is a valuable way for us to do that. Many of those who have used the *Unofficial Guide* travel books write to the authors to ask questions, make comments, or share their own discoveries and lessons. For lifestyle *Unofficial Guides,* we would also appreciate all such correspondence, both positive and critical, and we will make best efforts to incorporate appropriate readers' feedback and comments in revised editions of this work.

How to write to us:

Unofficial Guides
Macmillan Lifestyle Guides
Macmillan Publishing
1633 Broadway
New York, NY 10019

Attention: Reader's Comments

The *Unofficial Guide* Panel of Experts

The Unofficial Guide editorial team recognizes that you've purchased this book with the expectation of getting the most authoritative, carefully inspected information currently available. Toward that end, on each and every title in this series, we have selected a minimum of three "official" experts comprising the "Unofficial Panel" who painstakingly review the manuscripts to ensure: factual accuracy of all data; inclusion of the most up-to-date and relevant information; and that, from an insider's perspective, the authors have armed you with all the necessary facts you need—but the institutions don't want you to know.

For *The Unofficial Guide to Cosmetic Surgery,* we are proud to introduce the following Panel of Experts:

Dr. Saul Hoffman   Dr. Hoffman is clinical professor of plastic surgery at The Mount Sinai School of Medicine. He has been board-certified in plastic and general surgery since 1964, and has been in private practice in cosmetic and reconstructive surgery since that time. Dr. Hoffman was chief of plastic surgery at The Mount Sinai Hospital from 1982 to 1988, and at Beth Israel Medical Center from 1979 to 1988. He is currently chief of plastic surgery at

Beth Israel North Division in New York. Dr. Hoffman has written several book chapters and many scientific articles, and is currently in private practice in New York City.

Sue Augustine   Ms. Augustine is known internationally as a conference speaker, author of the extraordinary book, *With Wings, There Are No Barriers... A Woman's Guide to a Life of Magnificent Possibilities,* and a contributing author to the best-selling *Chicken Soup for the Woman's Soul.* She appears regularly on television and radio talk shows and has produced personal-discovery programs on audio cassette. Ms. Augustine presents over 100 informative and high-energy keynotes and seminars each year, helping women overcome the barriers of a negative body image, low self-esteem, and the emotional turbulence that results.

Dr. Paul R. Weiss   Dr. Weiss is certified by both the American Board of Surgery and the American Board of Plastic Surgery. He has maintained a private practice in Manhattan for over 20 years with a fully equipped surgical facility certified by the AAASF. Dr. Weiss, who is Clinical Professor of Plastic Surgery at the Albert Einstein College of Medicine, is a past president of the New York Regional Society of Plastic Surgery. He has been elected to the American Association of Plastic Surgeons and is active on numerous committees of the American Society of Plastic and Reconstructive Surgeons, including its Spokesperson Network.

Introduction

Every month or so, one of the major television networks broadcasts the results of a presidential popularity poll. My favorite popularity poll, however, is one that was featured in *Psychology Today*. It revealed that 60 million Americans don't like their noses. Thirty million don't like the way their chins look. Six million have a problem with their eyes; another six million dislike their ears. Me? I always want to change the last sentence I wrote.

When I first became a reporter, a seasoned writer told me the best investigative trick any beginner reporter can learn: Find the true insider's track, and people will tell me what I need to know. Insiders know the best scuttlebutt—where the best action is and who the true players are.

That's how I became interested in cosmetic surgery. I have a friend, Johanna, who is so fixated on cosmetic surgery that she is a veritable insider. She knows the scams, how deals can be cut, and when certain prices are negotiable. Johanna understands inventive methodologies better than several surgeons I've interviewed for various beauty articles.

The more I write about cosmetic surgery, the more surgeons, patients, psychiatrists, beauty experts, and dermatologists contact me about amazing discoveries. I've learned how savvy surgeons can spot (and diplomatically turn down) a "golden negaholic"—a super-wealthy prospect who will never be happy with his or her appearance regardless of the procedures done. I've also found out that patients who are "infomaniacs" (like my friend Johanna) can be very desirable candidates. These patients *have* to know every aspect of the procedure. In some cases, it almost appears that talking about the surgery is more exciting than the final results. Many infomaniacs ask for their own videos of their procedures! They are remarkably happy about the whole process and generally love their improved appearance.

The Unofficial Guide to Cosmetic Surgery is your VIP pass to the inside track on cosmetic surgery. Each chapter is filled with tips, secrets, and expert knowledge gleaned from thousands of true cosmetic surgery insiders. It's an expensive world. It is peopled by high-powered personalities. And, while there are scam artists and nightmare stories, there are many success stories, brought about by the great number of wonderfully dedicated and talented surgeons and doctors out there.

Today's Gold Rush: The Cosmetic Surgery Boom

A medical writer friend conducted a qualitative study of women and men in their thirties who have had cosmetic surgery. Completed in the spring of

1998, the study revealed that nearly 100 percent of the 300 respondents believed their cosmetic surgery made significant positive changes in their lives. Both men and women noted an immediate and perceptible rise in self-esteem in the workplace. Nearly all reported an increase in daily energy. Several other plusses appeared remarkable—being able to sleep better and feeling less anxious. Perhaps these cosmetic surgery results don't make riveting headlines; but I'm sure each patient interpreted his or her delightful results as great news.

In the last five years, cosmetic surgery technology has made quantum leaps. New drugs, improved monitoring techniques, and better anesthesiology options have, in some instances, diminished the sting of pain and lengthy recovery. In Chapter 4, for example, we give you the state-of-the-art developments in anesthetics. The good news? The debilitating nausea associated with several types of popular anesthetics has been diminished significantly. We know undergoing anesthesia is one of the more feared aspects of surgery.

Did you realize that most plastic surgeons don't administer the anesthetic themselves? They need to focus on the surgery, so they employ someone else to do the job. Chapter 4 tells you how to verify that your surgeon is providing you with the services of the best possible anesthesiologist or Certified Registered Nurse Anesthetist, commonly known as CRNA.

Many newer approaches involve less invasive methodologies and yield better results than those of just a few years ago. In tumescent and UAL liposuction, for example, current healing time is truncated by weeks for many prospects. And larger amounts of fat can be removed, too.

While the field of cosmetic surgery has made huge leaps, the process of exploring options hasn't been made easier. The process of finding the best surgeon—which we explore throughout the book, but particularly in Chapter 3—has not been made any easier. It's a common pitfall for novices to select a methodology before talking to top surgeons who can detail both the upside potential as well as the downside limitations of that approach. This book details why you should seek out expert names first and find out what each doctor suggests before deciding on the methodology (we give you a rundown on the most popular methodologies in Chapter 6).

Additionally, the nation's current cosmetic surgery boom has delivered a much younger market than just a few years ago. Today, adults in their thirties and forties are undergoing such procedures as facial liposuction, brow lifts, and laser removal of blood vessels and tiny wrinkles. From 1981 to today, the incidence of cosmetic surgery has increased nearly 70 percent. No longer reserved for wealthy dowagers, cosmetic surgery's biggest demographic group consists of adults 49 years of age or younger. Teens are another fast-growing segment. Together these groups account for nearly three-quarters of all cosmetic procedures performed today.

Since there is such a vast array of information about cosmetic surgery available today, you really do need an unbiased guide to navigate this complicated, costly, and booming field—and *The Unofficial Guide to Cosmetic Surgery* is it!

Traveling the Information Highway

As the increasing number of cosmetic options seemingly double each year, the average person must struggle to become more informed. And much of the newly emerging information can contradict facts and trends that were considered infallible in the early 1990s.

For example, phenol peels, once revered as the best way to deliver baby-smooth skin and remove sun damage, have fallen into disfavor in some medical communities. Anecdotal and clinical evidence of phenol-related scarring and uneven skin pigmentation has tarnished the methodology. Now, however, some of the nation's leading surgeons are reintroducing their modified and improved state-of-the art version of the phenol peel. And what about an AHA peel? Is that possibly better than laser resurfacing? Will a minilift rejuvenate your face and have you back on the job within a couple of days? More important: Is there *really* such a thing as a "minilift"? This book tells all.

Perhaps you believe that, without the guidance in this book, you can find a reputable hospital and trot through the process unscathed. Getting ripped off can't happen to cautious you. You won't take any chances. You might even have your surgery performed at a landmark hospital, where over the past 130 years the esteemed doctors have won 56 Nobel Prizes among them.

But, in fact, such a hospital in New York City was the scene of an outrageous cosmetic surgery scandal that continues to startle insiders by its troubling breach of accepted protocol. Here's what happened: A surgeon in training—a resident who had not completed his education—was found to be performing cosmetic surgery procedures on the sneak, having patients pay him in cash. It all came to light when one of his patients developed a hideous infection after a procedure.

What's in This Book (and What's Not)

While *The Unofficial Guide to Cosmetic Surgery* covers all sorts of state-of-the-art treatments for improving one's appearance, all of these procedures are elective, meaning *you* request them and *you* pay for them. Generally, there's no insurance coverage for cosmetic surgery, something we discuss in Chapter 2. This book does not cover reconstructive surgery per se. Repairing a serious birth defect or helping a cancer survivor adjust to their reclaimed life are best served by reconstructive or corrective plastic surgery performed by plastic surgeons.

This book is about aesthetics, the most common concern of patients seeking cosmetic surgery; so this book—and its tone—deal directly with elective surgeries that, for the most part, are simply cosmetic. These are procedures that modify some aspect of your appearance; many of the operations covered by this book have the potential to boost your self-esteem or help you regain an aspect of your body lost to childbearing or aging.

Is Cosmetic Surgery an Option?

Do you sometimes wonder if cosmetic surgery really is right for you? (If you're not sure, check out Chapter 1, in which we discuss other nonsurgical options that you can explore.) This book shows you how to get to the pit of your motivation. Chapter 1 gives you the insights of top surgeons, image experts, and even psychiatrists who explain candidly what cosmetic surgery can do for you—and what it can't.

There are trigger events that often spark an interest in cosmetic surgery— being teased as a teen, getting a divorce, losing a job promotion. Our insiders show you how to evaluate your motivations, health, and age, and put all of these in perspective with your financial situation.

Cosmetic surgery isn't cheap! Still, there are ways to save money. Before scheduling any consultation, simply ask your surgeon's receptionist if the initial consultation fee ($100 and up) can be deducted from your surgery. Almost everyone says yes! Or you might consider having some procedures done at a teaching hospital where fees may be significantly discounted and where you will be operated on by "students" but carefully monitored by seasoned hospital chiefs whose reputations are practically legendary. Other hospitals may discount cosmetic surgery clinic fees if you are willing to have a seasoned resident perform the procedure under the supervision of an experienced plastic surgeon.

The more you explore cosmetic surgery, the more you realize why the whole process involves a series of choices. We give you a list of key things to review and show you the meaningful points to consider in Chapters 3 and 4. Then you can individualize this *Unofficial Guide* list by adding variables that are important only to you. In this way, you'll walk away from your initial consultation with all the information you really need to make a smart choice.

You Call the Shots!

Armed with the many tips we give you in this book, you'll be able to comb through brochures and medical articles and cleverly separate the glamour of overinflated promises from the truth. Yes, the doctor is board-certified and a member of the Cosmetic Aesthetic Medical Society. Gee, you think, he must be good! Sure, he's a great *gynecologist*—which is the field he specializes in—a fact you'd never uncover unless you call the ABPS credential hotline (1-215-587-9322) that we tell you about in Chapter 3.

Before surgery, there are a number of personal considerations many doctors fail to mention—which we'll tell you about in Chapter 4. For example, if you're getting a face lift, *do* have your hair colored several days before surgery, because you won't be able to have it done for more than a month afterwards! And don't put your bare necessities high in the medicine cabinet if you're having pectoral implants. You won't be able to lift your arm up to reach them for a good week.

Pectoral implants? Yes, men represent one of the fastest growing segments in cosmetic surgery. Ten years ago, 1 out of every 10 or 12 cosmetic surgery patients was a man. Now, nearly a third of all patients are men (Chapter 8 is devoted to men's cosmetic surgery considerations). And, in some competitive metropolitan markets, men can make up nearly 40 percent of some surgeon's practices. Why? As Dr. Stephen Grifka explains, "Men like to compete and remain vital in the job market. Cosmetic surgery can be a simple approach—maybe just a neck lift—for a man to hold onto his job longer."

The stigma once applied to vanity and having cosmetic surgery is pretty much gone today. And with this book, you can learn how insiders also take the "sting" out of the process. Whether you're considering your first cosmetic procedure or are a veteran of several procedures, you'll find *The Unofficial Guide to Cosmetic Surgery* an invaluable resource. We wish you well on your journey to a renewed sense of self-esteem and happiness!

Planning Your Surgery

Chapter 1

GET THE SCOOP ON...
Determining whether cosmetic surgery is right
for you ▪ What motivates us to have cosmetic
surgery? ▪ What cosmetic surgery can and can't
do ▪ Some tough questions to ask yourself ▪
Exploring nonsurgical options

PART I

Is Cosmetic Surgery for You?

In New York City, high-powered baby boomers, including both men and women, represent nearly 70 percent of all cosmetic surgery patients—about 137,000 patients annually. No longer reserved for movie stars and wealthy dowagers, cosmetic procedures are being adopted by varied demographic groups. But is aesthetic surgery right for you?

Before opting for surgery, you must closely examine your true motivation. This chapter asks questions only you can answer: What's really bothering you about your looks? Does childhood teasing still haunt you? Are you worried that coworkers appear younger, sharper, and more energetic than you?

Personality and behavior style are also critically important to the success of any cosmetic surgery. We'll see how many prospects have behavior styles that tend to produce high levels of patient dissatisfaction. Key health issues and lifestyle considerations are explored here, too. We'll also look at an insider's screening device developed with the help of dozens of top cosmetic surgeons and psychiatrists who understand the complex dynamics of body image. Determine if your expectations are realistic. You may very well decide—as have many people I've known—that cosmetic surgery is not for you. I'll also discuss some nonsurgical options that are worth exploring.

No such thing as normal: what motivates us to have cosmetic surgery?

If your temperature were 98.5 degrees, would you swallow an erythromycin pill or jump into an ice tub to reduce fever symptoms? Probably not. So why are you contemplating cosmetic surgery? Sure, you may want to have that facial birthmark—a pesky red blotch the size of a postage stamp—removed. But that birthmark, like cauliflower ears, W. C. Field's nose, and a truly flat chest are normal. They're as normal as 98.5 degrees.

You've probably seen the craggy face of movie actor Edward J. Olmos whose award-winning performances include *Stand and Deliver*, among others. His heavily pockmarked skin is no different than that of Academy Award–nominated star James Woods. What we call bad skin, although normal, hasn't kept either actor (or the ever-evolving Cher) from pursuing major screen careers. Yet, despite how normal some physical traits actually are, adjectives used to describe them are painfully graphic. Most phrases are cruel: a backside as broad as a barn, hairy as an ape, face like a troglodyte, ears like a bat. Okay, so somewhere along life's reality path, maybe there is an ironic fork in the road: Most travel the average looks path. And some of us feel like we'll never get off the "average ugly" trail. (To add to the irony, appearance standards for the sexes remains considerably biased. Who can name a man who is said to have piano legs?)

How do you measure up?

Appearances help us manage human interaction. Physique, clothing, and face tell us gender, age, socio-economic status, emotion, and perhaps even character. When you meet another person, the psyche undergoes an immediate comparison. How do you measure up? It's part of our innate response to gain a psychological advantage over the other person, a secret ranking if you will.

Physical attractiveness can be your best asset, or it can be a liability. How much your own looks actually influences your daily life defines your motivation for wanting cosmetic surgery. While motivations vary widely, they either fall within the realm of normalcy or they exceed boundaries that most experts identify as unrealistic.

How do your motivations compare to those of other typical cosmetic-surgery candidates? For example, are you the person who rarely thinks about looks? Well rarely, that is, until recently? And now, in the last year, you're beginning to notice certain signs of aging: a chin that wobbles, even when you're not speaking? Or perhaps you're a 35-year-old business associate with a wonderfully successful career. Everything is pretty good in your life. Still, that potbelly has not budged one inch despite long hours on the gym's tortuous gauntlet. As long as these nagging concerns have not rendered you powerless, then thinking about your looks in these terms is natural.

However, when negative thoughts begin to influence your daily performance, causing you to hold

> 66
> In the simplest of terms, men and women considering cosmetic surgery want the same thing: greater peer acceptance. This also applies to teens as well as to older folks. Beyond this basic desire is an endless stream of individual desires, unique and mysterious as a person's fingerprints.
> —Dr. Sherrell Aston, New York City plastic surgeon
> 99

back and not deliver according to your potential, the power you ascribe to looks may be somewhat exaggerated. In truth, you may be motivated by goals that cannot be realistically addressed through cosmetic surgery. Quite possibly, following the post-operative period, should your expectations not be met, you might experience increased frustration.

Attracting the opposite sex is often a common motivation for considering surgery. Women worry about bosom size. Men? Thinning hair and penis size. It's no surprise that many of these image concerns go back to childhood where we learned values. How old were you when you discovered that the world around you—family, friends, perhaps even teachers—placed considerable importance on good looks? Maybe you were never taught that. Congratulations! You've avoided one of life's great snares that even cosmetic surgery can't save you from: valuing looks as the true measure of a person's being. So, if looking good at any cost played a significant role in your early development (or continues to be a prominent factor), proceeding with cosmetic surgery may only heighten any feelings of self-doubt. In particular, if an image problem has continually hindered you from developing healthy, intimate relationships that endure, your sense of self-worth may be best strengthened through psychotherapy. In these cases, and those that concern an inferior sense of sexuality, dealing with a qualified image psychotherapist prior to exploring cosmetic surgery will help you align your expectations with the potential results.

In broad terms, there are two opposing sides for wanting cosmetic surgery. To see which side of the equation you're on, let's examine random, everyday feelings of unattractiveness that we all experience. The often-mocked, bad-hair day is an example. Or imagine yourself as a fast-track marketing executive who has just muscled through an exhausting but highly successful four-hour client presentation. Before the presentation you looked great, but stress has taken its toll. During the break, you head to the nearest wash room to freshen up. Look in the mirror. Sure, go ahead and scream like Macaulay Culkin in *Home Alone.* That's fine, especially if you feel that your face is as wrinkled as your linen suit! For the remainder of the day, however, if you enjoy no sense of accomplishment—your looks are too troubling to you—your expectations may go beyond the range of normalcy. Why? In this made-up example, you did great! Your presentation was an enormous success. But you, rather than enjoying and savoring the victory, are permitting negative thoughts about your appearance to detract from your hard-earned accomplishment.

Can exaggerated hopes be overcome? Dr. Debbie Then, a San Francisco psychotherapist who specializes in image esteem, offers an answer. "Cosmetic surgery is not a panacea. It's a simple tool that has three key components. No matter how a person switches these elements around, an aesthetic procedure can only do so much."

Let me list the three elements of cosmetic surgery that Dr. Then continually emphasizes. They are so simple most people dismiss their significance:

■ Cosmetic surgery is an aesthetic, nonessential procedure.

■ Any surgery, cosmetic or not, involves some risks.

- At best, cosmetic surgery adds a boost to one's self-esteem and can improve one's appearance.

Did you notice that Dr. Then omits money from her equation? She explains, "Some people feel money buys anything. Their motivation takes on fantastic elements—maybe a divorce won't go through." A procedure may lift your spirits and help you feel more confident, but it won't necessarily change your life. Having liposuction alone won't snag you a promotion. You may feel more confident and assert yourself more positively at work, and that may *lead* to a promotion. But by itself, cosmetic surgery doesn't guarantee any life-changing benefits.

When cosmetic surgery does not deliver the desired results, disillusionment and bouts of depression often follow. In some people, such dissatisfaction triggers a string of other unsuccessful procedures.

The best candidates for cosmetic surgery

Personality and behavior play significant roles in the success of an individual's results. Personality says who we are. We might be perky or ponderous; at a given moment, you might be both. Generally, personality types who tolerate change well make the best patients. Extreme perfectionists, depressed people, negative people, and people with obsessive tendencies or controlling behavior all tend to fare poorly.

So who are you? And how would somebody who knows you really well describe you? As you read through the following four groups who do well with cosmetic surgery—I call them aesthetic value seekers—see if you can spot a few similar traits. However, first grab a piece of paper and write down three or four qualities that you think describe your general demeanor. Do it now. Don't try to wing it and keep key features in your head; actually write

Watch Out!
Cosmetic surgery junkies are prospects who are persistently dissatisfied with cosmetic surgery results. Their original appearance eventually is so radically altered, that their own identity is totally obscured. Rarely does cosmetic surgery provide relief or comfort, even when followed by extensive psychiatric counseling. Most face-lift junkies are women, but anyone can experience this addiction.

them down. Now write a sentence or two describing your basic lifestyle. How do you relax? Do you pay attention to your diet and cope well with stress at work? What things do you do to socialize? How do you typically interface with coworkers and the public in general? Make a few notes, then see if you can spot several shared traits with the following groups:

- *"I'm okay."* We all know people with a balanced self-image who tend to interact well with others, even if they are extremely reserved and quiet. Their daily lives are varied. Emotional outbursts are rare. They do not fear spending time alone, nor are they phobic about social gatherings. They are members of some community—a workplace, family, or the town in which they live. These types may be bothered by a physical characteristic that they would like to improve or change.

> **"**
> Oh, I'm so inadequate. And I love myself!
> —Meg Ryan, American movie star
> **"**

- *"I'm okay, but . . . "* The line between this group and the former is almost imperceptible; both share many similar traits. However, for this group, the bothersome feature gains psychological importance over time. Fat thighs, for example, keep them from going to the beach with friends. Occasionally, they may perceive rejection when there is none. This low self-esteem, however, does not govern their daily lives. After cosmetic surgery, the majority enjoy good results. Their adjustment may be slower; building confidence usually involves time.

- *"I'm okay, but help!"* Invariably this group is made up of teenagers or young adults. They have a particularly high awareness of an appearance flaw. These defects may be real or imagined. For some, their looks seem to have changed overnight. Protruding ears, a disproportionate nose, or bad skin begin to erode self-esteem. When teasing and ridicule ensue, the young person's confidence may not adequately develop. Cosmetic surgery can prevent the emotional turmoil brought on—whether real or imagined—by the rejection of others.

- *"I'm okay, but I love my corporate earning power!"* For the most part, "baby boomers" refers to the sizable demographic group born during the two decades that followed W.W.II. Despite their previous mantra, "Never trust anyone over thirty," a number of boomers have slipped comfortably into middle age. They are proud of their role in the sixties social revolution while enjoying 21st century technology. These cosmetic surgery candidates achieved significant career success early on. Now an equal number are keen on staying at the top; they view cosmetic surgery as a tool to help extend corporate tenure. They wish to look polished, rested, and in shape. And in the wake of corporate downsizing, cosmetic surgery is their corporate survival tool.

Unofficially...
The United States Census Bureau estimates that nearly one in four people will be 55 years or older by the year 2000. That's the largest increase in this age group since the beginning of time. However, this group will be the first seniors to stay exceedingly fit and have more cosmetic surgery than previous 50-year-olds.

Health and lifestyle considerations

There is no risk-free, easy surgery. Your general health and lifestyle dictate how well you heal, even more than a dream team of surgeons can. Be prepared for glitches. Possible complications include excessive bleeding, a severe reaction to the drugs, or infection. You may end up with a scar you never dreamed possible. Even with simple surgery, a blood clot can form and travel to the lungs. Statistically, of course, complications such as these are rare. But your general health and lifestyle deserve scrutiny.

Not everyone is an automatic cosmetic surgery candidate. Obviously, certain existing conditions—diabetes, lung disease, heart trouble, high blood pressure, and other chronic conditions—can be unacceptable risks to some patients. A number of these variables can be carefully evaluated and accommodations can be made on an individual basis. It's important to be completely honest with your doctor. Don't withhold information or try to influence his or her decision.

Also, while some diseases or chronic conditions won't prevent your having cosmetic surgery, your final aesthetic results may vary somewhat from the norm. Being overweight and out of shape place extra stress on your heart. Smokers and heavy drinkers have special considerations. No aesthetic surgeon will proceed with a prospect who smokes unless the person guarantees to abstain for two weeks (or longer, for patients undergoing face lifts) prior to the surgery. Abstinence must also continue for another ten days to two weeks postsurgery.

A vitamin C deficiency curbs the healthy production of collagen, the protein substance that begins production about four days after injury and clusters to fill in the defective area for weeks thereafter. It was observed in W.W.I that wounds failed to close unless fresh foods containing vitamin C were eaten. Later experiments proved that the speed of healing and strength of scar tissue are directly proportional to the vitamin C intake. About 4,000 milligrams of vitamin C daily can take care of average healing needs.

Skin that has been exposed to radiation also heals poorly because small blood vessels are often damaged; these small vessels help carry white blood cells, antibodies, and other substances that promote healing.

Watch Out!
It's not just the billows of cigarette smoke that are bad for your skin. Nicotine is the real culprit, creating havoc as it washes through your blood. Many surgeons report that nicotine ingested during the pre- and postoperative period can lead to raised scars that are worse than normal and take far longer to heal.

Frequently we underestimate the effect that daily stress places on our well-being. Signs that you may be suffering more stress than you realize can be identified by answering "No" to one or more of the following questions:

- Do you fall asleep easily?

- Do you pay bills and deal with personal finances without feeling stress?

- If your job causes fatigue and creates stress, have you developed remedial ways to offset their toll, such as taking short breaks throughout the day or not bringing work home over the weekend?

- Are the things you truly value in life being realized?

- Do you generally feel good about your job, family, and friends?

- Do you have a stable, satisfying relationship with an intimate partner?

All of us probably have a fair idea about what constitutes a healthy diet and which routines invariably contribute to a robust and sound lifestyle. For the purposes of cosmetic surgery, certain foods, habits, and stress factors wield a great impact on your ability to heal normally. The following test helps you to evaluate your body's lifestyle and healing capability in very simple terms.

More than three negative answers to any of the following questions indicate that your current diet and low-level exercise routine may compromise final results and lengthen the normal healing period.

- Do you make exercise a part of your regular daily routine, such as taking the stairs rather than the elevator, or taking an after-dinner walk?

- Do you participate regularly in a sport such as swimming or golf?

- Do you restrict sugar, saturated fat, and salt in your daily meals?

- Do you drink less than five ounces of alcohol (no more than three drinks or four or five beers) weekly?

- Do you include healthy amounts of fiber in your diet and limit your intake of red meat to less than three times weekly?

- Do you limit your caffeine to the equivalent of two cups of coffee or less a day?

- Do you eat or drink out of boredom or in response to some frustrating situation?

The insider's body analysis

Welcome to the *Unofficial Guide* Health Spa. True, it's Spartan, but like many of my recommendations, it costs nothing. And the upside potential is enormous. I'm pretending we're at a spa for a specific reason. As you undergo this unique body analysis, imagine, if you can, that you look your best. Don't fixate on a chipped manicure or feeling exhausted. Hands and feet have been pampered and you've gotten plenty of rest. In fact, your hair and appearance have been successfully made over by a top image consultant.

In the next room, a team of body image specialists will help you evaluate the type of cosmetic surgery you're considering. Working together, you need to complete a Body Analysis Checklist.

You will be asked to rate your appearance, using four choices. As you assess the following body areas, assign one of the following four letters to each:

Timesaver
Many of our daily routines are so second nature, we take much for granted. To scrutinize yourself more thoroughly, buy a small pocket notebook devoted only to your cosmetic surgery exploration. Carry it with you at all times, entering medication concerns to ask your doctor about and jotting down questions as they occur to you.

- *Neutral (N)* means you feel indifferent toward that body part.
- *Positive (P)* means you really like a body part and value its appearance.
- *Negative (N)* means you don't like a body part.
- *Disturbing (D)* means you wish to surgically alter a body part.

BODY ANALYSIS CHECKLIST

Lower body:

1.	Feet _____	
2.	Ankles _____	
3.	Calves _____	
4.	Knees _____	
5.	Other: _____	

Thigh and midsection:

6.	Thighs _____	
7.	Lower abdomen _____	
8.	Waist _____	
9.	Buttocks _____	
10.	Other: _____	

Upper torso and extremities:

11.	Chest _____	
12.	Back area, general posture _____	
13.	Hands _____	
14.	Arms, especially upper limbs _____	
15.	Other: _____	

Face and head:

16.	Neck and face in general _____	
17.	Chin and jaw line _____	
18.	Mouth _____	
19.	Cheeks _____	
20.	Ears _____	

21.	Nose _____
22.	Eyes and eyelids _____
23.	Brow _____
24.	Forehead _____
25.	Complexion _____
26.	Hairline and scalp _____
27.	Other: _____

Here's how to score your responses:

For every N (for either *Neutral* or *Negative*) or P answer, give yourself 10 points. Add your total and write the amount here: _____.

For every D answer, give yourself –15 points. But before tallying your D entries, go back to each D and ask yourself these critical questions to make sure that body part really rates that response:

▪ Is this feature a true obstacle to your enjoying life right now? If yes, keep the –15 entry.

▪ Does this feature hold you back from achieving certain goals, deprive you of getting close to others, or limit you in other meaningful ways? If yes, keep the –15 entry.

Put the total score for all D entries here:

_____.

Now add the two totals and put that number here:

_____.

An overall total of 200 points or higher suggests a healthy acceptance of your appearance.

What areas stood out in your responses? How do you feel about your size? Is your weight just fine as it is? Would you like to lose five or ten pounds, or do you want to lose 30 pounds or more? You should be aware that obese people (those who are about 20 percent over the average weight for their frame) are not good candidates for cosmetic surgery because the excess weight affects the overall condition of their health.

Are you a yo-yo dieter or a person with an eating disorder, including anorexia? Those prospects with eating disorders are also not good candidates for cosmetic surgery, and it's likely that, like obesity, this condition will negate a cosmetic surgeon from accepting you as a patient.

Finally, if you have some *D* responses, you may be ascribing too great an impact to the successful outcome of any cosmetic surgery procedure. Making a change to your appearance is more about your perception of what the change can accomplish for you rather than the reality of the change itself.

What surgery can and cannot do

Patients who like their cosmetic surgery results appear to enjoy an almost immediate improvement in self-confidence. Invariably this translates to a greater interest in social activities, and men and women alike express a greater hope about the future. In personal relationships, women note a higher incidence in declaring their needs more readily. Realistically meeting the demands of others becomes easier and less daunting for many women. As one Chicago 33-year-old television producer phrases it, "I now sulk less when pressure hits. I'm able to work through awkward situations that I previously felt incapable of handling. I always felt people were staring at my acne scars." Both married and single women note a significant satisfaction in sexual activities. Men, too, experience an almost immediate surge in self-esteem. Many feel they are more likely to take career risks and note a higher comfort level in dealing with the opposite sex.

> **"**
> In the 19th century, attaining the beautiful female body required wearing a corset, which led to difficulty in breathing, constipation, weakness, and a tendency to violent indigestion. Unfortunately, women's bodies have always been viewed as unfinished or in need of decoration through carving, incision, tattooing, and other disfigurement.
> —Susan K. Ward, psychotherapist and director of the National Eating Disorder Hotline and Referral Service
> **"**

Regarding career challenges, many describe an ability to compete better. One Atlanta architect notes he is less likely to bully others. "It sounds horrific," he recalls, "but being out of shape with my big gut somehow triggered outbursts on the tennis court. My body did not respond the way it used to when I was younger. So my tennis partner got the brunt of that anger." Nearly all happy postop patients, from teens to octogenarians, cite a general increase in energy and well-being.

The list of what cosmetic surgery can't do is endless, but the four most common disappointments include:

- Depression and low self-esteem have not abated.
- Hopes and personal desires were not met.
- Pain, recovery, and healing time were greater than expected.
- Pain and healing were not worth the costly investment.

In reality, the majority of cosmetic procedures are successful. Most patients claim they would repeat the entire process without hesitation. However, while the percentage of patients who are disappointed with the results is low, if you're one of the very unhappy patients, personal frustration and a sense of defeat are 100 percent.

Key questions to ask yourself

When you're initially trying to decide whether cosmetic surgery is for you, it's natural to feel uneasy or anxious. You might even imagine disastrous results. All of these thoughts are perfectly fine. Altering our appearance represents a frightening breach of our original identity. Since the beginning of time, this

Bright Idea
Have you ever had your hair dramatically styled or cut significantly shorter? How did you react? If you took it all in stride, good for you. Such behavior shows some healthy adaptability. However, many cosmetic surgery procedures produce permanent results. If you've made no change to your appearance in a decade, ask yourself if you're flexible enough to handle cosmetic surgery.

fear has been examined in troubling tales and disturbing folklore. Even today, primitive masks displayed in museums can cause the average person to feel some vestige of alarm. Again, apprehension is understandable as you undergo this internal process. You may want to slow down and do some serious thinking, however, if you experience virtually no apprehension, and expect to sail through the entire process without a second thought.

Questions from surgeons that trigger patient anxiety are often answered wrong. The incorrect response is not deliberate, and most prospects don't intentionally lie. They simply can't face the ramifications of what an honest answer might compel them to do. Here are some of the areas that often signal emotional hot points. It's worth exploring in greater detail the most complete response you can give to these questions.

Have you assessed the risks, both major and minor?

Ask yourself, "Will the surgery (or implants) create a problem that doesn't already exist? How will I cope with unexpected results?" Patients who easily dismiss the potential risks are often the most surprised and anxious when even minor complications develop. What will you do if your initial results seem undesirable? Surgery can play havoc with finances and work schedules. Ask yourself if you're being unrealistic about financing your surgery. Does your schedule allow for an adequate recovery period? Explore the possibilities of how your body will react. Never let the surgeon assume all the responsibility; participate in planning your procedure.

Are you hiding your plans from loved ones?

You may adore your results, but a loved one, particularly a spouse, who is not informed about your planned cosmetic surgery may feel alienated and become highly critical of your new appearance. Yes, it's your body. But if you fear discussing your plans with others (family and close friends), how will their disapproval affect you? Cosmetic surgery patients who deliberately hide their plans are often the same people who thrive on lavish praise. They are very needy of another's approval. Ask yourself who you do not want to tell, then try to figure out why.

Are you considering surgery to please others?

Undergoing surgery to please someone else invites disaster. There's a higher risk for future psychological problems. Be completely honest: Are you trying to please another person rather than please yourself? Is the surgery designed to boost a flagging relationship? Are you hoping to attract more attention? A common example is the ambivalent wife who, with some misgivings, proceeds with breast implants to please her husband. Many such patients experience ongoing distress years after the surgery.

Other questions to ask yourself

Were you inspired to have surgery because a broadcast news item piqued your interest and you've done your own research about the possibility? Do you know someone who has talked about having a similar procedure and was candid with you about all aspects? Do you know anyone who had cosmetic surgery who can recommend several doctors? Are you willing to accept the possibility that the results may not be exactly what you envisioned? Do you accept the responsibility for electing this surgery?

Nonsurgical options

So much has been written about eating well that most people feel only a monumental change in eating habits, accompanied by Olympian exercise, will

Timesaver
It's a good idea to bring a friend to your initial consultations with surgeons. Having someone with you not only reduces stress, he or she is more likely to remember key questions you may overlook and later recall what details were covered. And during recovery, a buddy can help with ice packs and handle those ordinary tasks you think you can manage, but really can't.

produce enormous benefits. This is simply not true.
A few small changes can yield significant results to
your health and appearance.

Diet

We all know it's better to avoid lots of saturated fats,
red meat, butter, and cream. But you need not
exclude these foods from your diet all the time. Try
doing the right thing 80 percent of the time, and a
few slips aren't likely to condemn your overall effort.
A balanced diet simply means taking food from as
many different sources as possible. Here are several
healthy diet quickies practically anyone can fold into
their daily eating routine:

- Eat plenty of raw, fresh fruits and vegetables,
  such as celery, carrots, peppers, apples, pears,
  and oranges.

- Drink at least six to eight glasses of water a day.

- Add more fiber and roughage to your diet, such
  as brown rice, whole-grain bread, potato skins,
  fresh parsley, and strawberries.

- Skip creamy dressings and rich sauces.

- Cut back on sugary foods and baked goods
  made with processed ingredients; these are
  highly caloric and contain little or no nutrients.

- Eat dinner four hours before you go to sleep;
  keep the last meal light and on the small side.

Exercise

How hard is it for you to get up and do something
fun? Do you need a change? If you're feeling mildly
blah or blue, simple exercise can hoist you out of
your slump. Your new exercise program need not
be arduous or painful in order for you to reap the
rewards. Simple walking is one of the best ways to

Moneysaver
Many nutrition-
ists claim that
drinking more
water can plump
the skin, encour-
age better diges-
tion, and
encourage renal
and lower tract
functions, all of
which add
sparkle and
shine to skin,
eyes, and hair.
Remember, only
water is a pure
hydrator;
caffeine is a
diuretic. Before
opting for
expensive and
perhaps unnec-
essary proce-
dures, try drink-
ing more water.

improve your body and psyche. Doing less rather than more yields a higher success rate. Over-achieving in the early stages is a surefire way to fail. Also, daily exercise may help alter brain chemistry, giving you a lift. Once exercise is continued on a regular basis, healthy brain chemicals, notably endorphins, are more readily produced. The muscular and cardiovascular system respond positively, too. In sum: *You begin to look and feel better.*

If you lead a sedentary life or are at least 25 pounds overweight, always consult a doctor or qualified fitness expert before beginning any exercise program to determine what kind of exercise would be best for you. To prevent injury, warm up and cool down afterward. Stretch as often as you think of it. If you feel dizzy, breathless, or experience any pain, stop exercising immediately.

If you answer "Yes" to any of the following questions, consider beginning an exercise program immediately:

- After running to catch a bus, are you out of breath?
- Is walking up three flights of stairs an effort? Do your legs ache, even slightly, when you reach the last flight?
- After sitting on the floor, is getting up difficult?
- Does tying your shoelaces or picking up something on the floor require some straining on your part?

Any addition of simple exercise into your daily routine will deliver meaningful benefits. Park your car at the end of the parking lot each day when you drive to the office. Carry your groceries to the car rather than using the cart. Take a stroll after lunch and dinner. Take the stairs instead of the elevator. When you wake up, stay in bed and stretch. Even small changes can make a big difference.

Image consultants

Most Fortune 500 corporations know the value of image consultants; practically all executives who are being groomed for top management slots are sent to the best image gurus. Men and women undergo complete makeovers. Along with a new diet and exercise program, why not consider hiring an experienced image consultant to revolutionize your appearance? How to dress, walk, talk, and present yourself with confidence are skills that can be acquired. If you can positively change how you think about your appearance, the positive behavior of others toward you will also improve.

The Association of Image Consultants International (1-800-383-8831) has a wealth of experts who specialize in various areas, including appearance, styling, speech, and color analysis. Ask for the names of several consultants in your area so you can compare costs and services. It's important to find someone who matches your taste and budget. Also be aware that the quality of image consultants can vary widely—it's best to ask for references so you can check with other satisfied clients.

Therapy

66
No one can make you inferior without your consent.
—Eleanor Roosevelt
99

You can achieve a lasting personal change without having to invest thousands of dollars and hundreds of hours on a psychiatrist's couch. There are many psychotherapists who are qualified to resolve a number of esteem issues using short-term cognitive therapy. If you have defeating thoughts about your appearance, you will feel and act as if there is little hope.

Through psychotherapy, you may discover that specific negative thoughts about your appearance actually relate to a totally separate matter. A Denver psychiatrist recalls helping a world-renowned engineer come to terms with a startling realization. The patient's introversion and extreme shyness, *not* his appearance, held him back in social situations. Top in his field, the engineer simply lacked the basic social skills to relax and chat casually with associates and friends. The more he worked on people skills the less he worried about his appearance.

Developing other benchmarks and standards beyond the superficial aspects of appearance provide meaningful, satisfying, and enduring levels of self-worth. Several books, notably Naomi Wolf's *The Beauty Myth* (Anchor Books, 1991) and J. Rodin's *Body Traps: Breaking the Binds That Keep You From Feeling Good* (William Morrow, 1992) also provide useful insights.

Deciding what you can live with

There are many appearance concerns you may choose to live with. One of the more liberating epiphanies comes with the knowledge that some things you can change, and some you can't. Many issues about looks are simply not worth the worry. In other words, fiddle, if you must, with those areas you can improve, and ignore the no-win situations.

To successfully embark on any changed behavior strategy, engage in a course of action that makes you feel good about yourself. When you're having negative thoughts, act in a way that turns your bad feelings around. Treat yourself: Buy that Hugo Boss suit that really flatters your physique. Distance yourself from any circumstance, even highly critical people, that triggers bad feelings. Develop simple

Unofficially...
Many celebrities have made a physical imperfection their trademark: Consider Barbra Streisand's nose, Jay Leno's chin, Cindy Crawford's mole, or the gap in model Lauren Hutton's front teeth!

affirmations that you can easily recall and say them daily. Record your own tape of positive self-talk.

Write down personal goals and find ways, however small, to include some aspect of these aspirations in daily plans. Living your goals rather than dreaming them is the best way to achieve self-confidence!

Just the facts

- Cosmetic surgery is a personal choice best shaped by realistic expectations that must be weighed against the risks.

- Your individual level of satisfaction and general recovery is largely determined by your own hopes, personality style, self-esteem, lifestyle, and health issues.

- Take responsibility for developing a realistic agenda of what you want altered, and evaluate your decision in context with what top surgeons and other aesthetic medical experts recommend.

- Keep your hopes pragmatic and your desires practical.

- Cosmetic surgery is not for everyone; other options, including diet, exercise, psychotherapy, and accepting the terms of one's appearance, can deliver equally effective results.

GET THE SCOOP ON...
Assessing the risks that all surgery entails ▪
Financial considerations: surgery, anesthe-
siology, and hospital fees ▪ Insurance coverage
issues ▪ The special considerations of men,
African-Americans, Latinos, and Asians ▪
Teenagers: The growing youth segment seeking
cosmetic surgery

You've Decided That You're a Candidate . . . Now What?

Okay, you've done your homework and read the previous chapter, and you think you might be a candidate for cosmetic surgery. Now what? First, understand that there are special considerations for each sex. For example, men tend to have coarser features, so subtle alterations may translate less noticeably to the male body. Females with very delicate features require extremely precise modifications.

Minorities have special considerations, too. As the minority economic status continues to rise, many African-Americans, Latinos, and Asians seek to enhance their appearance through cosmetic surgery. The medical field is increasingly populated by skilled surgeons who offer many splendid ways to achieve a natural, appealing look that respects the ethnic integrity of each person.

Apart from special considerations for men, women, and varied ethnic groups, the burgeoning

Chapter 2

25

field of teenage surgery has created its own set of variables and pitfalls. There are other factors you need to look at also, such as your age and health, the cost of the procedure, and insurance coverage.

This chapter stresses the need to individualize your search. No matter who you are, if you read this chapter you'll know exactly what to do.

Basics to consider

In the past, anti-aging candidates tended to opt for rejuvenation somewhere around the 50-year mark. Today, however, the field is wide open. A man may have perfectly legitimate reasons for having cosmetic surgery on his eyelids or under the eyes at the age of 35. No amount of sleep will alter the bags under his eyes; perhaps his look of fatigue is simply genetic. In other words, your age (and sex) no longer dictate when you get a face lift. If your appearance bothers you and something about your looks intrudes on your self-esteem, then it's time to think about making some changes. I interviewed one plucky great grandmother who simply got rid of a few wrinkles so that her face matched how young she felt! She was always an active person; now she is just a bit zippier than before. Hardly anyone viewed her as old at 81 years. And no one seems to notice that a few wrinkles have vanished. But, as she put it, "I wanted a pep tonic and that's what cosmetic surgery did for me."

Research has shown, though, that self-esteem is not improved by cosmetic surgery but requires inner transformation as well. Patients with a poor self-image often see no significant changes after surgery and are thus disappointed. Self-esteem issues must be dealt with prior to surgery.

Age and lifestyle don't preclude certain risks

Each candidate must continually assess the degree of risk for his or her procedure, taking into account age and lifestyle issues. There are three basic risks that can occur with any candidate, regardless of age or health. Be sure to discuss the possibility of each with your doctor:

- *Bleeding.* A certain amount of bleeding is expected with any procedure. Any black and blue marks you've had in the past have resulted from bleeding under the skin. However, in surgery, excess bleeding under the skin can accumulate and require an additional procedure to eliminate the excess. Be sure to discuss bleeding and bruising with your surgeon prior to the procedure so you are better prepared.

- *Infection.* Despite the extreme care taken to prevent it, becoming infected is a gamble that varies with the type of procedure performed. Incidents are rare, and antibiotics prescribed as a preventative measure before, during, and after reduce this risk dramatically. But it can happen. If you smoke, take steroids, or have certain vascular conditions, you may run a higher risk of becoming infected. Discuss this with your doctor before proceeding.

- *Sedation complications.* Mild sedation induced by a pill or the more powerful tool, general anesthesia, are numbing devices that permit surgeons to cut and repair the body. There is the potential for a serious reaction. Some patients complicate the sedation process by not being absolutely honest with the doctor about medications or certain mild medical conditions.

Unofficially...
Hematoma refers to a pooling of blood or the formation of a blood clot that is localized. Hematomas can occur with practically any surgery. Should you experience localized bleeding in a delicate or vulnerable area, in some cases the final aesthetic result may be compromised.

Remember, your doctor is not your parent. He or she will make no value judgment. It is essential that you give your doctor your true age and complete medical history. Anesthetic glitches can run the range from mild nausea to abnormal heart rhythm. And without a complete, honest approach you are inviting danger.

Elective means expensive

Cosmetic surgery is not cheap. Be prepared—your insurance company likely will *not* pay for anything. For example, many basic surgical fees do not cover the following:

- Hospital stay
- Medical tests and photography
- Anesthesia

Almost without exception, cosmetic surgery must be paid for by you. And most surgeons will ask for full payment of the surgeon's fee prior to the operation. It's a basic of elective surgery: You want it, you pay for it up front.

It also is a reasonable protection for surgeons. Imagine the jittery patient who appears to listen intently to everything the doctor tells her prior to the operation. However, she really hears nothing! Her memory fails to recall how bruising and swelling will compromise her appearance during the initial postoperative stages. When she finally sees herself, she panics and refuses to pay the surgeon.

Along with the surgeon's fee, it's quite possible you may have to pay for another highly skilled doctor: the anesthesiologist. Their fees can run from several hundred dollars upward to thousands of dollars. And hospitals, too, are costly: An overnight stay or longer may be required. Many cosmetic facilities have arrangements with local banks to help patients finance elective surgery.

As an individual, you must weigh the advantages of making monthly payments versus creating a significant burden with such an arrangement. There are three costs one should anticipate when exploring cosmetic surgery. Possibly you'll have to pay for only one, but be prepared. The first cost is for *surgery*.

The average surgeon's fee has a slide factor that travels from downright low, up to the lofty and beyond, on to the stratospherically high. It is simply not a universal truth that "You get what you pay for." You can pay $10,000 for a face lift and feel it is worth every penny. Or you can pay a huge sum and see few results. The following table lists the approximate costs for the surgeon's fee only, covering a variety of procedures.

Watch Out!
Cosmetic surgery can run into the thousands of dollars, which often comes out of your pocket. Insurance companies are increasingly aggressive about refusing any medical cost elected by the patient. Avoid surprises: Find out what your insurance will cover *before* you have the surgery.

SURGEON'S FEE, BY PROCEDURE

Surgical Procedure	Average Cost
Breast augmentation	$2,784
Breast lift	$3,224
Breast reduction	$4,877
Male breast reduction	$2,419
Buttock lift	$3,319
Cheek implants	$1,930
Chemical peel	$1,513
Dermabrasion	$1,536
Collagen injection, per 1cc injection	$281
Ear surgery	$2,262
Eye surgery—Both uppers	$1,580
Eye surgery—Both lowers	$1,622
Combination uppers and lowers	$2,775
Face lift	$4,407 ($4,783)*
Forehead lift	$2,275 ($2,494)*
Laser resurfacing—Full face	$2,556
Laser resurfacing—Partial	$1,191

Surgical Procedure	Average Cost
Liposuction, any single site	$1,710
Nose reshaping	$3,104
Thigh lift	$3,336
Tummy tuck	$3,795 ($3,832)*
Upper arm lift	$2,539

*Denotes use of endoscopy. (Source: American Society of Plastic and Reconstructive Surgeons)

Remember, fees mean nothing by themselves. You have a lot of homework to do when it comes to selecting your surgeon, which I'll discuss in Chapter 3. The fees in this table, however, represent a national average and in no way do they suggest the amount you may end up agreeing to.

The second cost you may have to bear is for *anesthesia*. There are as many as 30 million anesthesia procedures performed each year, according to the American Society of Anesthesiologists. Anesthesiology tools include approximately 26,000 anesthesia machines at a basic cost of $50,000 per device. Expensive, yes? That's one of the reasons why cosmetic surgery is so costly.

Like many medical specialties, the field is constantly seeking ways to refine technique and equipment. For example, there's a computer-controlled system for delivering anesthesia, which developers claim reduces postoperative nausea to almost nil. The system uses a computer microchip to calculate precise dosages. Because the system bypasses use of a respirator, it is said that the patient wakes up very clearheaded but with no nausea, no vomiting, and no nasty taste in the mouth.

Another major cost you may also have to absorb is for *hospitalization*. Indeed, many procedures can be done on an outpatient basis. But it is often not

Unofficially...
In the United States, there are roughly 30,000 professional anesthetists. These include anesthesiologists who are physicians specifically trained in this field. Also, there are nurse anesthetists. These are registered nurses who are nationally certified in anesthesiology. Discuss with your surgeon how your sedation will be administered.

the procedure alone that dictates this. Your health, lifestyle, age, and other issues must be evaluated by your doctor. The procedure may be simple, and all of your research may suggest that having breast implants done in the morning will have you home in the afternoon. But if your surgeon anticipates certain reactions or complications, you may have to spend the night in the hospital. This can easily cost several hundreds or thousands of dollars.

Even the insured must pay

The best way to determine if you qualify for some coverage is to read your individual insurance policy and carefully check your benefits manual. When it comes to reimbursing you, insurance carriers will evaluate your claim based on the primary reason for your operation. They will want to know if the operation is being done *primarily* to provide relief of symptoms or for aesthetic reasons, only. If there is one whit of vanity at issue or any cosmetic concerns, the insurance company will likely deny your claim. On the other hand, procedures such as breast reduction or reconstructive surgery with cosmetic components may be covered.

To see if you might receive the maximum you deserve, ask your primary care physician to provide you with documentation of your need for this procedure. This must be done *before* you decide to proceed. A pre-authorization letter written by your primary physician to your insurance company *prior* to the operation can often answer whether or not you're covered.

Remember: Doctors can tell you what is *not* covered, but many are vague about what *is* covered. Relying on verbal assurances or secondary sources who assure you that your claim will be honored, can

Bright Idea
There are ways to sedate patients that eliminate (or significantly reduce) the chance of nausea. These anesthetics are called *non-emetic*. Discuss this option with your medical team if you have a history of queasiness.

Moneysaver
A pre-authorization letter, prepared by your primary care physician and sent to your insurance carrier, should explain the procedure in detail and ask for a written confirmation that you are covered and what your benefits are. The level of coverage will be sent to either you or your doctor (make sure you request a copy).

be a costly mistake. If your doctor seems vague about this issue, head for the door.

Here's a case in point: Consulting a friend whose mother's sister is a surgeon who straightened the nose of a cousin who had some trouble breathing and had the whole procedure—valued at $12,000—totally reimbursed should set off an alarm. Don't become swept away by the excitement. You may hear only the things you want to hear. So, indeed, you may qualify for insurance coverage. But be prepared to battle the odds. Be prepared to battle your insurance carrier.

On the off chance that your carrier will share the expense, be sure to have this information available when you first consult your doctor:

- Group plan number
- Policy number
- Insured's social security number (and yours, if the insurance is in the name of your husband, wife, or parent)
- Insured's name
- Insured's employer
- Your date of birth

Be certain to grasp every detail about coverage before you have surgery. If you have any questions, spend time with your benefits representative who should be qualified to answer any issues you have about iffy areas.

Some cost-sharing options include:

- *Deductibles*. In this instance, the carrier requires that a certain amount of medical expenses be paid by the patient before the insurance company initiates coverage.

Watch Out!
If you find a physician who is willing to fiddle with your form so you get reimbursed, run from his office! Clearly, such a physician will also lie to you as well.

After your deductible requirement is met—
most range from $100 to $500 on average—the
carrier will then pick up 75 percent or more of
covered medical expenses. Remember, you still
must pay the percentage the carrier doesn't
cover.

- *Co-payments.* Flat-rate co-payments require the
  patient to pay for a defined share of covered
  medical costs which varies with each policy. The
  insurance company then is responsible for the
  balance.

- *Percentage-based co-payments.* These are much like
  regular co-payments. However, rather than paying a defined rate, the patient is obligated to
  pay a percentage of covered medical costs. Your
  carrier will then pay the balance or fixed
  amount based on your policy.

Scheduling your surgery

Once you've clicked with the surgeon of your
choice, be prepared to nail down the surgery date.
Many surgeons are booked weeks or months in
advance. Others often maintain a few openings
within their busy schedule.

First, the time of year could have a major impact.
I was intrigued to discover that America's cities during the glittering December holiday season often
become crowded with cosmetic surgery candidates.
If you've had enough with grueling travel plans,
unending family obligations, and the notorious holiday "blues," this may be your year to give yourself a
much deserved present. But, as this chapter points
out, don't forget: There may be several return trips
to the doctor's office. So if you're coming from out
of town, you'll need to stay for awhile, and it's

unlikely you'll be able to drive yourself. Plan to have a backup plan, especially if an ice storm strikes.

Foot surgery, for example, is often best left to the warmer months when wearing sandals speeds recovery. Following dermabrasion, the skin should not be exposed to bright light for several months. So, if you're a tennis buff and can't imagine giving up your weekly game, you must appreciate that neither sunblock nor a wide-brimmed tennis hat will save your newly abraded skin.

Eyelid surgery and face lifts are sometimes followed by incredible swelling and unusual bruising. I can think of two avid skiers who rarely bruised after catastrophic falls; yet each blew up like eggplants following conservative face lifts. That means if there's a key social event—your best friend's wedding, a graduation, or a special trip—you must allow ample recovery time to accommodate looking your best.

In many cases, some cosmetic procedures don't really settle in until the first anniversary. I find that many successful eye jobs still have a wan look for six months or so following the procedure.

Second, don't forget to allow time for tests and many small details that can take hours, such as filling out forms and waiting in line for medical tests. You may have to schedule X-rays and blood workups even if you enjoy perfect health. Plan to have professional "before" photographs taken; your physician will recommend a good photographer (your doctor will take a set of before and after photographs as well). Sure, go ahead and schedule the photo shoot before work. But not a wisp of make-up is allowed. The photographer will pull your hair back and place you under bright lights. If you have an important business meeting following the

Timesaver
If you have selected a very busy surgeon who is booked heavily in advance, nail your date down quickly. If you'd rather not wait the several months some doctors require, ask if you can be notified of any cancellations. If another patient is forced to cancel, frequently the switch still allows you enough time to get comfortably ready.

photography, allow time to freshen up. In other
words, be prepared to invest more time than you
imagined. And then tack on a few extra weeks as
well.

You can't hurry time

There is nothing quite so individual and unpre-
dictable as each person's own healing period. The
importance of a healthy postoperative weight cannot be exaggerated, so watch your weight loss and
weight gain vigilantly. Having a face lift and then losing 15 pounds can compromise your results dramatically. If careful dressing changes are required
following surgery, you must make arrangements to
have a family member or nurse help with such care.
Any dependency problem, including alcohol, will
create havoc with healing.

Time for wound healing is really a matter of
months, not days or weeks. And in many cases, the
level of pain and distress is greater than the patient
imagined. A typical face lift will preclude you from
engaging in any form of exercise (other than walking) for one month. No aerobics, no simple
machine work at the gym. You won't be able to lift,
bend, or strain. "Great," you say, "I'll finally get my
desk cleaned up!" But simple things such as tidying
your sock drawer or making lists may be canceled by
waves of fatigue. You probably won't be able to see
clearly enough to address an envelope, let alone get
caught up on those overdue thank-you notes or dis-
organized recipe cards. If you want to schedule little
jaunts, remember: For many procedures, you will
not be able to drive a car or take an airplane for 10
days or longer. Staying put and not going back to
work, even for the most antsy type, is part of the
healing process.

Get by with a little help from your friends

No matter how capable you are, be forewarned: You will need support and all kinds of help. Many men imagine they will slip through the process with the skill of James Bond. It doesn't quite happen that way. You may decide not to tell certain people. Fine, but telling no one and going it alone is dumb. Try, if you can, to get over any perceived stigma attached to your operation. Don't feel guilty. And stop thinking that cosmetic surgery is a luxury reserved for the wealthy. Ask for help.

Part of the support phase is figuring out before surgery what you are going to say to people about your absence. Perhaps you'll want to "throw them off" by mentioning that you're going away to a spa? Or do you plan to say nothing? You really have only three options. Here's what you can choose to do:

- Make an excuse or tell a lie.

- Say nothing.

- Mention something about your pending procedure.

However, *now* is the time to weigh the plusses and minuses of each scenario. Choose one. Do it now—before surgery!

And one caution: If you opt to lie to everyone, it requires a lot of "emotional" work and the ability to remain consistent. As an example, let's say you're going for liposuction, and to explain your absence, you tell everyone you're taking a cruise down the Nile. Fine. Just be able to answer those everyday, innocent questions that people toss your way just to make idle chatter. How was your trip? Was the food any good? And you may find yourself forever having to recommend the best places to stay in Luxor. Or

Unofficially...
The majority of cosmetic surgery candidates have a household income of $50,000 or less, not what most people would consider wealthy. Patients who do well with cosmetic surgery feel they have nothing to hide and know how to ask for support.

name that special prescription that kills pesky amoe-
bas in the local drinking water.

In sum, only you can decide if it's appropriate to
share the information, if any, about your cosmetic
surgery plans.

Special needs of men and minorities

As cosmetic surgery attracts a greater number of
men and different ethnic prospects, procedures are
streamlined to address specific aesthetic needs.
Historically, the true beneficiary of cosmetic
surgery has been one group: women, notably
Caucasian women. For this reason, the field already
has expert techniques for enhancing many female-
specific anatomy needs. But more and more men
(currently almost 30 percent of all patients having
cosmetic procedures) and ethnic groups are seeing
the advantages of cosmetic surgery.

Male considerations

I devote Chapter 8 to the special considerations for
men when it comes to cosmetic procedures, but let's
touch on them here. For everyone, there is often
the perception, true or not, that an older executive
may be less up-to-date and less efficient. It is this
concern that is attracting so many male prospects to
cosmetic surgery. Since many of the same procedures are used for both sexes, the basic technique
may vary very little. However, each sex has its own
considerations.

With men, any scarring that may occur may be
more difficult to hide within the facial area. To correct a double chin or jowly neck, liposuction alone
may correct the problem for younger men. But
older candidates may require a full neck lift. With
the latter procedure, the platysma muscles that run

Watch Out!
If you want to
pretend to be
sick for a week
or two, it's your
decision. But
if you take the
"flu" route,
be prepared
for friends con-
stantly checking
in on you. And
how did you get
over that hideous
flu and some-
how look
stupendously
younger?

down each side of the neck may have to be tightened. These muscles tend to be thicker in men (and do not typically pose a greater challenge to experienced surgeons), so care must be taken to disguise the incision.

For example, due to the presence of facial hair, men have a richer supply of blood to the face. Typically men bleed more during surgery and are more likely to develop hematomas, the temporary pooling of blood under the skin, which can occur after surgery. But for both men and women, any incision in the temple area requires great skill.

Peels and the like tend to strip away the surface of the skin; a number of male patients told me they were unprepared for the swollen appearance and bright pink skin color. This sunburned appearance lasts for several weeks. Alcoholic drinks can flush the complexion; you may have to forego the cocktail hour for a month. Men who are programmed to be stoic and work-driven are not the best candidates to take it easy for the recuperative time necessary. And studies show that men feel foolish asking for help and are likely to develop postoperative depression unless they can call upon some support or coping mechanism. So, discuss with your surgeon how you can beat the blues on your way to a new look.

Aesthetics for Latinos and African-Americans

Thankfully, the trend in all cosmetic surgery is toward naturalness. The tight-as-a-balloon face lift has vanished along with the ridiculous worship of the Great White Idol. A good surgeon will try very hard to preserve ethnic features that are in harmony with an individual's overall appearance. Both Latinos and African-Americans must be skeptical of surgeons who are known for a specific look. Strict

Bright Idea
Many men actually like a scruffy beard's ability to camouflage incisions and recovering skin. Also, be prepared to grab a cap before you go outdoors. And slather on sunblock as your surgeon advises.

adaptation of any typical Caucasoid feature is likely to do a disservice to the balance of any face. A one-size-fits-all design tends to disrupt facial harmony and look artificial.

The normal features of whites, Latinos, and African-Americans—indeed, many ethnic groups—are remarkably different. Each has its own unique standard of true beauty. The best surgeons respect these ethnic variables and know how to adapt them for each person. African-Americans and Latinos should seek a surgeon who is sensitive and extremely qualified at interpreting what their desires and specific needs are.

Ethnics are well advised not to defer to a surgeon's recommendation without engaging in healthy dialogue about how the recommended change will truly enhance his or her ethnic character. Surgeons who specialize in minority considerations should be able to demonstrate through references, sensitivity, and an impeccable track record that she or he is capable of translating and rendering what is best for the patient as well as what the patient wishes. I advise everyone to remember a truth about the exceptional surgeons: The ones who are true leaders, the brilliant innovators in their field, will not perform "a look" that goes against their aesthetic values.

As aesthetics for minorities are championed by leading surgeons, there is a growing agreement as to what constitutes beautiful distinctions. For example, more surgeons seem to agree that an attractive African-American nose is often shorter in length and has a more rounded tip than a typical Caucasian nose. It can also be wider than the distance between the eyes and still be considered aesthetically pleasing. In some cases, the best change is a subtle one for the alteration to be aesthetically accurate, and ethnically appropriate.

Whether repairing the upper eyelid or the nose to add additional height to the bridge, you and your surgeon must analyze your entire face and profile. It is a common mistake of some ethnic candidates to evaluate only the area that is being modified. If your doctor can provide it, ask to see a sketch or computer image. While it won't give you a completely accurate picture, you'll have some idea of how the proposed change will create harmony with your entire appearance. If a sketch is unavailable, ask to see before and after photos of similar candidates. To a great degree, all cosmetic surgeons, especially those who work with minorities, must represent a unique amalgam of a renaissance artist—both a portrait interpreter and sculptor of the beautiful things that make each of us unique and desirable.

Many surgeons interested in ethnic cosmetic applications have begun to redefine what needs fixing. In the past, doctors might have tried to narrow the bottom of broad nostrils and end up overcorrecting the nostril base. In extreme cases, a triangle with a fold at the top of the nostril formed; this undesirable look is called "notching." Now there are better ways to narrow the base so that nostrils taper with a soft, curved edge. One surgeon, Ferdinand Ofodile, a Manhattan-based Nigerian cosmetic surgeon, has catalogued the various noses he's worked on as Director of Plastic Surgery at Harlem Hospital in New York City. He's identified three types of African-American noses:

- African, with a wide, fatty tip and a relatively low bridge

Unofficially...
The standard of beauty in today's society has long been Caucasian. In the average black magazine, models may have some African-American features but, for the most part, they have long, narrow faces and narrow noses. However, this standard appears to be changing in favor of more diverse looks.

- Afro-Caucasian, with a cartilaginous tip and a raised bridge

- Afro-Indian, with a fatty tip and a hump on the bridge. Dr. Ofodile hopes this catalogue will make it easier for surgical residents to make sense of diversity and avoid disasters.

Apart from features, doctors are increasingly sensitive to the differences of how each skin type might respond to cosmetic surgery. Darker-skinned adults have a greater chance of developing a problem with scarring or pigmentation change. For these candidates, finding a skilled surgeon specially trained in minority skin characteristics (and who understands each person's healing ability) is essential.

Interpreting the almond eyes and high cheekbones of Asians

Culturally, Asians appear less concerned than Caucasians when it comes to the natural aging process. Thus, face lifts among this ethnic group tend to be rare; to diminish mild signs of aging, some Asians are more likely to favor chemical peels. Scarring tends to show more on Orientals or East Asian skin; incision placement is critically important and requires great sensitivity. Creating a crease between the lashes and the brow—called double-lid surgery—is the most popular procedure for Asians. Understandably, the procedure to remove the epicanthic fold has drawn criticism. Many doctors believe they have to remove this fold to make the eye wider—a bigger eye is what most Asian patients request. But some skilled surgeons suggest simply manipulating the muscle and tissue of the lid to make the lashes turn upward—Asian eyelashes usually point down. This adjustment can create an

Watch Out!
Most Caucasians are born with a crease in the upper eyelid, but only half of all Asians are. Asians have a special fold, called the *epicanthic* fold. This unique feature creates the almond-shaped eye so wonderfully characteristic of Orientals. Adapting a strict interpretation of the typical Caucasian places the crease too high on Asians, imparting a permanent startled look.

illusion of larger eyes with very little trauma. Asians with an unusually flat and broad nose may wish to give greater definition to their profile. But there is rarely a desire among today's East Asians—either here or abroad—to westernize their appearance. Their desire is simply to improve an aspect that is consistent with their ethnic beauty standard.

On a qualitative basis, I have observed that the motives behind cosmetic surgery appear to differ between Asian and non-Asian women. When the Oriental woman considers cosmetic surgery, if she was not American-born, it is often at the encouragement of her husband, and she does so with the desire to please her mate. On the other hand, it is not unheard of for the American woman not to tell her mate. I know of dozens of examples of American wives who have chosen simply to surprise their husbands after the fact.

Apart from the appearance of eyes, two other distinct Asian features are the roundness of the face and high cheekbones. A good aesthetic surgeon understands that the integrity of these features should not be compromised. And since Asians often have characteristically broad noses, the combination of these three factors creates a sense of flatness. Therefore, Asians who explore cosmetic surgery should carefully consider how subtle dimensions might be added to the face while maintaining their standards of balance and beauty. Asians, like minorities and all prospects, should seek a total look that is aesthetically pleasing.

The burgeoning teen segment

In the late '90s, there were roughly 15,000 reported cosmetic surgery procedures performed each year on teenagers. That's about 2 percent of all cosmetic operations and most of these consist of nose jobs, breast and ear alterations.

I feel strongly that not every teenager seeking cosmetic surgery is well suited for the operation. Without emotional maturity and an understanding of what cosmetic surgery can change, results—short and long term—can generate dissatisfaction. Teens must finish growing and maturing before even considering cosmetic surgery; bone structure often does not begin to mature until 18 years or older.

Peer pressure plays a significant role in the teenage years. Indeed, we all want to fit in. But getting a nose job just because your best friend got one is not a good reason to have the procedure done. Also, as a teen matures, many begin to value their own unique characteristics. There is something to be said for keeping what is yours alone.

Well-intentioned parents need to fully understand what the young adult is seeking, and why. Many surgeons and professional organizations suggest parents consider three factors when discussing cosmetic surgery. These topics can help evaluate how healthy a teen's concern truly may be:

- *The teen initiates the request.* While parental support is essential, the teen's own desire for a cosmetic improvement must be clearly expressed and repeated over a period of time.

- *The teen has realistic goals.* The young person must appreciate both the benefits and limitations of cosmetic surgery, avoiding unrealistic expectations about life changes that will occur as a result of the procedure. Also, the teen should have respect and appreciation for how costly a procedure can be.

Unofficially...
Teens are usually similar to adults in their motivation and goals; but changing an attribute too early can compromise a person's identity. What a teenager views as physically attractive can change within a matter of months. With teens more than any other group, prospects need to grasp that any cosmetic change may become a lifetime decision.

- *The teen demonstrates an appropriate maturity.* Does your son truly understand the levels of pain and healing involved? Will your daughter be able to handle the ugly phase of healing when an area looks almost disfigured? Clearly teens who are prone to mood swings or erratic behavior, who are abusing drugs and/or alcohol, or who are being treated for clinical depression or other mental illness are not candidates.

Many a young adult suffers the agony that severe acne eruptions cause. Some of this may be brought under good control by the proper use of modern prescription drugs, such as Retin-A. In addition to supervising the use of these medications, cosmetic surgeons or dermatologists may be able to improve acne scars by smoothing or "refinishing" the skin with a laser or with a sanding technique called dermabrasion. This, however, should be done only when the acne has abated.

If it is decided that cosmetic surgery is an option for the teenager, both the parent and teen should find the best surgeon who has a great deal of experience with young adult patients. All should confidently agree that the teen's physical maturity has peaked. If not, changes to the nose, ear, face, and general anatomy may overcorrect an area, delivering a result that is likely too small and out of proportion once the figure matures.

Just the facts

- All surgery entails some risk, regardless of your age or health.
- Take a close look at what your insurance carrier will pay, if anything. A pre-authorization letter written by your primary physician to your

insurance company *prior* to the operation can often answer whether or not you're covered for a procedure.

- Cosmetic surgery is expensive; fees are often due before the procedure.

- Schedule your surgery only after you've considered how much time off you can afford to take and who will help you manage your recovery.

- Men and minorities typically have special considerations that should be clearly understood by doctors.

- Teens need to mature physically and emotionally before surgery or the results may be out of proportion.

Proactive Strategies

PART II

GET THE SCOOP ON...
Tips for remembering all the details ▪ Elements
that make cosmetic surgery successful ▪
Financial considerations of cosmetic surgery ▪
The lowdown on medical boards and associations ▪ Investigating a surgeon's credentials to
find the one who is right for you

Making Truly Smart Choices

Chapter 3

The *Los Angeles Times* reported in a story late in 1997 that a Beverly Hills surgeon who specialized in laser surgery, Dr. Adrianna Scheibner, had her license suspended by the Medical Board of California when at least four patients underwent unsatisfactory treatment that left some of them with third-degree burns and permanent scars. The newspaper reported that one patient wrote a check for $60,000 after being medicated and underwent up to 20 hours of strong laser treatment over two days. The patient is permanently scarred.

The lesson? A glamorous zip code and piles of cash can still be worthless in the land of vanity. They can't guarantee high-caliber surgery. Unfortunately, there are plenty of medical charlatans who are willing to take your money in exchange for shoddy work. This chapter shows you how to develop meaningful leads for finding qualified surgeons. All practicing doctors have credentials. You need to understand which documentation, references, and recommendations are meaningful for you. If you can decipher the impressive letters that often follow a surgeon's name—such as Dr. Sleightofhand, F.A.C.S.—you're less likely to get ripped off.

I'll also show you how using a planning notebook will help you keep track of all the little details. How can you anticipate the budget for elective surgery? Again, if you don't want to be robbed or make an impulsive costly mistake, do some dollar work before. There's a lot to cover, so let's get started.

(As a postscript to Dr. Scheibner's suspension, she can, as can any doctor with a suspended state license, still practice in *another* state. Scary, huh?)

Planning a winning strategy

Rather than becoming overwhelmed by the prospect of where to begin, here's a strategy to get organized. Buy a small notebook (don't keep little sticky notes or scattered papers) and devote it to your search. Divide the notebook into five sections:

1. Preliminary items

2. Consultations

3. Surgery

4. Postoperative stage

5. Frequently called telephone numbers

This is your planning notebook. Use it to record your thoughts and remember details as you read through certain chapters. Plan on carrying it with you most of the time, not just when you're off to consult with your first surgeon. In the next chapter, you'll learn which questions to ask your surgeon; questions that fit your needs can be entered in the "Consultations" section. Write surgical details (such as what your doctor prescribes for your particular surgery, including a number of medical tests) in the "Surgery" section, along with items you'll want to bring to the surgery site. For example, if you're having a face lift, you should make a note to wear a shirt that can be buttoned in front, not a pullover sweater.

You won't remember every key name or number. There are dozens of details that pile up before and after the day of surgery. Even if you're happily looking forward to your new nose, stress places a burden on the brain, so record in your planning notebook every telephone number that you come across or use. Begin this step now. Keep every number, especially those you think you'll never need again, such as a hospital fax number or a medical board.

Your basic list will require several critical things you'll need to get done. Clearly, these too vary considerably for each person. However, considering the following eight general areas will help you get the planning process underway:

- Budget considerations
- Personal medical data
- Surgeon qualifications, certifications
- Surgery proposed by each physician
- Credential verification
- Surgery date
- Presurgery "to-do" list
- Recovery "to-do" list

Elements of a successful cosmetic surgery

There are several key things that contribute to a successful cosmetic surgery experience. Careful planning, accepting responsibility for your search, and

Unofficially...
Research has shown that most postoperative patients recall only one-third (or less) of the information their surgeon provides them before surgery. You can beat that average by keeping a planning notebook.

Bright Idea
Once you create a master list, make several copies. Then you can update your list every week or so as you tailor the process to your own needs.

not taking the easy way out (such as closing your eyes and pointing to a doctor's name in the Yellow Pages) are all steps you can take that will foster success. Keeping your expectations in line is also essential.

In the next sections, we'll discuss other ways you can make your cosmetic surgery experience a successful one.

Be open-minded

I know a sophisticated building designer who read a magazine article on dermabrasion. Right away she decided that was the procedure for her sun-damaged skin. Several top San Francisco surgeons tried to dissuade her from this particular methodology, telling her that what she needed instead was to remedy the *tone* of her underlying muscles. Eventually, though, she prevailed and found a willing new doctor. It was no surprise that her uneven results proved to be disappointing and her recovery was much longer than she dreamed possible.

Her narrow thinking and presumptuous attitude—not just the doctor's willingness and lack of expertise—underscore how any intelligent person can rush down the wrong path in the planning process. Given the many evolving methodologies, your personal needs and individual appearance variables, use this time for discovery. Let the doctor help you decide which methodology is best. Ask why. Then see if you agree. If you've done your homework, you should be able to tell whether the doctor is pushing new equipment or prescribing the best approach for you.

Know your medical history

Make a list of past surgeries you've had, no matter how irrelevant you may think each is. Maybe you

Watch Out!
In the early stages, as you read and become more knowledge-able, there's a risk of making snap decisions. One of the best ways to assure your success is to use the early phase as a genuine learning process.

had an appendectomy or had your tonsils removed. Write down any allergies. Make notes of things you'll need to tell your doctor. You'll find yourself adding to this list as you go through the research process. Keep a running inventory of prescriptions and over-the-counter remedies you take and know the dosage. Cosmetic surgery can bring on depression during the postoperative period. Now's the time to observe any mild mood swings so you're not caught off guard later. Record any headaches or pains you experience before surgery. In other words, *tune into* your body.

Avoid dangerous mistakes

Money is an important commodity, but time is also an important—and typically overlooked—commodity. The first mistake many people make is to race through the process. If you're near a major city and know several leading surgeons, it still may take six or eight months to schedule surgery. If you're a novice and know nothing about qualifying a good plastic surgeon, you may need several months just to narrow your prospects. Take out your calendar and decide when you can afford to take time off for surgery. Then allocate enough time for doing research to locate the best doctor, check out credentials, and schedule consultations. Don't forget time off from work to get to and from the doctor's office. For many people, just lining up each doctor and getting to the appointment and back takes an average of three hours.

Accept responsibility

I'll say it several times throughout this book: Cosmetic surgery is *elective*, meaning *you* make the choice. Don't abdicate responsibility. Make a plan and modify it if necessary, but don't cut corners.

There are several things that can really make your surgery go well and acting responsibly is one of them. No one else controls the amount of effort you put into the search and listening to what people tell you. Evaluate all information given to you. This is your job.

Don't mislead your doctor

I began this chapter by telling you the hideous tale of the flagrant mistakes of a Beverly Hills surgeon. One rarely hears, however, of devious patients who deliberately lie—covering up certain medical conditions or plans for recovery—thereby undermining the surgeon's plan of action or compromising healing. The best plans are based on honesty. Don't lie to the doctor about your age, medical history, or medical condition.

Don't spend money you don't have

There is something about cosmetic surgery that brings out the idiocy in people. Some prospects fantasize about a dramatic transformation and their reverie takes off like an action-adventure movie. Instantly they imagine themselves as a new (and very rich) person. They imagine liposuction or a nose job landing them a better, high-paying job. They picture themselves winning the lottery or attracting the super-wealthy spouse of their dreams. Like an auction that can sweep up a person of modest means into bidding fever, cosmetic surgery, too, can seduce you. Don't spend money you do not have. It happens frequently: A person considering one modest procedure suddenly signs up for a complete, unaffordable makeover. Going into debt to pay off the surgery can create horrible, unpleasant suffering and depression. Don't let the fever sweep you away.

How will I pay for cosmetic surgery?

At this point, you may wish to jot down how much expendable income you can afford or are going to invest, remembering, of course, that nearly all cosmetic procedures (and attendant expenses) are not refunded by your insurance carrier.

If you don't know how much your surgery will cost, check Chapters 7 through 14, which cover the average fees for varied procedures. The fees range from several hundred dollars to multi-thousands of dollars. Each doctor's consultation will cost about $100 and there are other fees, including medical tests, an overnight stay in the hospital, and anesthesiology. These are outlined in the next chapter.

Only you can answer if the medical costs are worth the personal investment. However, I do caution you not to go into debt for a procedure you can hardly afford.

Planning and budgeting

As a general rule, all cosmetic surgery fees are due and payable before surgery. Unlike some small-town dentists and other accommodating medical providers, most cosmetic surgeons don't let patients use an installment plan to fund the surgery. However, nearly all doctors and certainly all hospitals do take major credit cards. Before you decide to charge any expense, however, have a dollar amount in mind. Stick to this number. It's easy to succumb to a lot of little fixes that cost thousands of dollars which you charge on your credit card and—with interest fees—will eventually cost you double.

The following table lists what some typical fees actually cost when charged and repaid over five years.

Moneysaver
If money is an issue, tell the surgeon during your consultation. Ask if she can recommend less expensive options to fix what bothers you. Also, before going to a consultation, ask the doctor's receptionist if your consulting fee can be deducted from the surgery fee if you proceed. Most will say yes if a patient asks first!

Procedure	Typical Fee	Actual Cost When Charged and Repaid Over Five Years (at 18% Interest)
Nose job	$3,104	$4,660
Liposuction	$1,710	$2,567
Chemical peel	$1,513	$2,271

You may also wish to seek a bank loan to fund your surgery. Some doctors do have relationships with banks that can provide loan information and payment schedules. But keep a dollar amount in mind and don't exceed it. And remember, as with all bank loans, the money is advanced to you, you pay the surgeon, and repay the bank for the use of their money with interest.

Teaching hospitals

For many people, their income simply precludes them from exploring cosmetic surgery as an option. If this is your situation, look into teaching hospitals that offer cosmetic surgery clinics. You may have to demonstrate to the facility your inability to pay; frequently, a tax filing statement will suffice. Other hospitals, notably Manhattan Eye, Ear & Throat in New York City and Cedars of Sinai in Los Angeles, offer excellent, top-of-the-line surgery performed by doctors who are about to successfully conclude their surgery residency. (For a list of top teaching hospitals in the United States with cosmetic surgery clinics, see Appendix B.)

Residents have already completed many hours of plastic surgery. Typically these hospitals do have waiting lists; others will be able to operate within weeks if you are prepared to do so. Invariably, staff at all support levels are typically highly qualified and extremely professional. The medical pretesting requirements and surgery are highly regulated and supervised by top surgeons in the field. As a patient you will receive the same surgical attention (even more so, in some cases) as full paying patients who may pay up to ten times your fee. All postoperative attention is included. If you live near a major city, you are likely to find several top hospitals that offer this service. Check the public relations department of that hospital or speak with someone knowledgeable in administration.

A few cautions: Many hospital switchboards may not know what you are seeking, so persevere. If you know a top surgeon in your area, try checking his or her office to see if someone there can recommend a reputable teaching hospital. And, rather than sign up for several major surgeries, you may wish to try a minor procedure first. Also, undergoing fewer than three procedures at one time is often the best way for a novice to proceed, because you'll have a chance to see how your body responds to this type of surgery before you invest in any other procedures.

Look nearby for the best leads

If you live near a major hospital, one with an excellent reputation, call the operating room and get the name of the top anesthesiologist. Then call this doctor's office and ask for a plastic surgeon recommendation. Doctors who are in the operating room regularly often know who the top surgeons are. Friends and family members (or an acquaintance who may have had the same procedure you want) can also be good sources of information.

Here is a frightening reality you must revisit each time you decide to pull a name out of the Yellow Pages: Anyone with a medical degree and a license

Watch Out!
Never take a
referral at face
value. If some-
one suggests a
name, ask why
he or she recom-
mends the doc-
tor. According to
congressional
testimony in
1989 by Harvey
Zarem, M.D., a
past director of
the American
Board of Plastic
Surgery, well-
meaning family
doctors have
unwittingly
referred patients
to unqualified
surgeons.

to practice medicine can legally perform cosmetic surgery in the United States. Yes, that means you could find an obstetrician who also performs rhino-plasty. Therefore, should you get a recommendation from a contact in a hospital or from a friend whose sister is a nurse, evaluate the recommendation through satisfied patients, word of mouth, mutual hospital affiliations, or other forms of professional contact. Knowing a surgeon socially is not a recommendation. Ask instead, "Who would you send your daughter or husband to?" for rhinoplasty, lipo-suction, or whatever procedure you are considering.

If you get the name of a surgeon from a contact, see if you can find someone who has used this surgeon. Ask if that person is satisfied with the outcome. Would she have done anything differently? Would she use the same surgeon again? You may also ask the cost of the surgery at that time.

An operating room nurse or technician who assists surgeons or your county or state medical society can also provide leads. While professional medical societies don't recommend one doctor over another, they can provide a list of board-certified physicians who are members of their organizations. In addition to names and phone numbers, medical societies can tell you which hospitals and medical schools their members are affiliated with.

The American Society for Aesthetic Plastic Surgery offers a toll-free referral service: Call 1-888-272-7711. This service can provide names of *board-certified plastic surgeons* in your area who specialize in the kind of cosmetic surgery you want.

The Plastic Surgery Information Service can be reached at 1-800-635-0635. Operated by the American Society of Plastic and Reconstructive

Surgeons, it also provides names of *board-certified plastic surgeons* in your area and can determine if a surgeon you are considering is board certified. This credential is crucial to your decision process, as I'll explain in more detail a little later in this chapter.

You can also try a hospital physician-referral service. Naturally, this service will refer you to its own doctors. But hospital affiliation implies the doctor meets a certain level of education, training, and patient care. It further implies that the physician's credentials and work are subject to review by other doctors. But obtain referrals only from a major hospital with an impeccable reputation.

Deciphering a doctor's credentials

There is a simple way to weigh a doctor's credentials, but first you'll need to grasp a few basics. Here's an example to make my point: Let's say you see two ads for two doctors. Each ad offers various cosmetic procedures. Each doctor appears professional and both are board certified. The first doctor belongs to the Aesthetic Medical Society. The second doctor has several letters after his name: ABPS. Both doctors have practiced in the medical field for eight years. Both ads are slick, intelligent, and appear in separate leading national magazines.

Would you know the first doctor received her cosmetic surgery training at a week-long seminar held at a Caribbean resort? Might you guess that before the seminar, she was a pediatric surgeon? Of course not. But now she could be *your* "expert." If you understood credentials, you'd know the second doctor, who claimed ABPS (American Board of Plastic Surgery) membership, completed three years of general surgery, followed by two years of supervised residency in plastic surgery. That's what ABPS means

(I'll talk more about this and other organizations in just a moment). Of course, it's up to you to see if the ABPS claim is valid. I'll show you how.

Deceptive ads, deliberately misleading phrases, and empty memberships in important-sounding organizations are some of the artful tactics some doctors use to rip you off.

Unqualified doctors who deliberately mislead

Why are there so many "iffy" medical organizations that sound so impressive? First, the field of cosmetic surgery is lucrative, so it attracts doctors who wish to cash in on the demand and the newer, growing technology, although these doctors may not be the best qualified. Cosmetic surgery doctors keep just about 100 percent of the fees they collect. Some physicians have even set up their own organizations in order to lend a sense of legitimacy to their deceptive practices. You probably didn't know, for example, that the American Board of Cosmetic Surgery doesn't require a surgical residency. To belong, the physician must be evaluated by his peers and pass an examination. That pretty much makes it a self-designated, self-regulated board. Membership is open to doctors who practice cosmetic surgery—for example, gynecologists who perform liposuction—but they do not necessarily have to have the qualifications for membership in the American Board of Plastic Surgery.

Secondly, many prospects don't do their homework. Many of us put our faith in medicine because the field has the built-in reputation for helping people. You may think it is unusual to find a surgeon certified in some other specialty who does general cosmetic surgery. Truthfully, it's more common than you might imagine. Since many botched

Watch Out!
A 1989 government investigation concluded that cosmetic surgery was too frequently being performed by doctors who had no special training. If your doctor is affiliated with a hospital, see if he is authorized to perform the procedure at the hospital even if you're having it done in his office. That means he has the approved surgical expertise hospitals require of their staff. Also, should a problem arise, you can be transported quickly to that hospital.

cosmetic procedures do indeed involve a board-certified doctor, it's your job to ask, "Certified in what?" If the doctor you're considering has not completed a special cosmetic surgical residency, keep looking for a surgeon who is certified by the ABPS. (And remember, no matter how prestigious membership in the American Board of Plastic Surgery seems, it is no guarantee that your surgery will go off without a risk. But at least the surgeon understands the basic principles and has had the training to do the procedure.)

Although board certification is not a guarantee, it is one piece of evidence toward evaluating a surgeon. If the ABMS (American Board of Medical Specialties) does not recognize the board providing the certification, it is probably a self-designated board and is meaningless for you. In the following pages, we'll take a look at the credentials that are truly meaningful.

American Board of Plastic Surgery (ABPS)

The most important certification comes from the American Board of Plastic Surgery (ABPS). A physician who is board certified *in plastic surgery* has been certified by the American Board of Plastic Surgery, the official examining board for plastic surgeons. Holders of this certification are qualified to perform reconstructive and cosmetic surgery.

The American Board of Plastic Surgery is one of the 24 specialty boards recognized by the larger, overseeing board called the American Board of Medical Specialties, or ABMS. This larger board sets high standards of education, training, and experience.

To have a cosmetic doctor certified by the ABMS, which sanctions the American Board of Plastic Surgery, signifies several key criteria:

Timesaver
If you need information about a doctor's credentials, try calling his office. The receptionist or nurse may be able to tell you which hospital the doctor uses or what specific certification is claimed. Also ask for information about the procedure you are considering.

- The doctor has earned a degree from an accredited medical school.

- The doctor has completed at least three years of supervised general surgical training.

- The doctor served a two- to three-year residency training program in *plastic surgery*.

Residency training is viewed to be critically important because it includes both cosmetic and reconstructive surgery.

After at least two years of practice, the physician must pass comprehensive written and oral exams in plastic surgery before becoming board certified. This is not a rubber stamp; the failure rate is about 30 percent. Board certification in plastic surgery usually indicates the doctor is trained to do a wide variety of cosmetic procedures on the face and body. Like most rules, there are some exceptions. For example, nonplastic surgeons who perform cosmetic surgery may concentrate on the part of the body in which they already specialize. A dermatologist might learn to do laser peels to ameliorate facial wrinkles, or an ophthalmologist might seek training in cosmetic eyelid surgery. To me that makes sense. However, in my opinion, a gynecologist is not automatically qualified to perform liposuction on midriff, thighs, and buttocks just because the object of her specialty happens to reside in an area close by.

Through advertising, public relations, and credible-sounding organizations that smack of high-caliber plastic surgery credentials, you can be misled. Here's where the waters get murky. There are scores of other self-designated boards that set their own standards for membership. Be careful! These standards may incorporate some of the requirements

Watch Out!
A qualified head and neck doctor—a certified otolaryngologist—should do surgery on the neck and above only, not on breasts or other parts of the body.

of the recognized surgical specialties. Or they may require nothing but a warm body and a membership fee. (A list of ABMS-recognized boards appears in Appendix B.)

There are two other associations (not boards!) that are highly creditable, and membership in one or both can suggest that your surgeon shares the ethical principles and professional standards the associations set forth.

American Society of Plastic and Reconstructive Surgeons (ASPRS)

About 97 percent of this country's 5,000-plus board-certified plastic surgeons belongs to the American Society of Plastic and Reconstructive Surgeons (ASPRS), headquartered near Chicago. Only doctors who are board certified in plastic surgery are permitted to join and become active members. The ASPRS mission includes educating the public about plastic surgery, promoting high professional standards of care through its educational foundation, and lobbying government and insurers on behalf of plastic surgeons. Membership in ASPRS, or in any professional society, is voluntary.

American Society for Aesthetic Plastic Surgery (ASAPS)

A second association, the American Society for Aesthetic Plastic Surgery, Inc. (ASAPS), based in Arlington Heights, Illinois, requires members to be board certified in plastic surgery and to devote a significant portion of their practice to cosmetic procedures. Plastic surgeons must be in practice at least three years before they can apply for membership. In addition to providing information to the public, the aesthetic society's goals include promoting and encouraging the highest standards of ethical conduct and responsible patient care among its approximately 1,100 members.

American Board of Anesthesiology (ABA)

If you require an anesthesiologist, it is imperative that he or she be ABA board certified by the American Board of Anesthesiology. Once you learn your anesthesiologist's name, call 1-919-881-2570 to verify credentials and certification.

Many office procedures use nurse anesthetists who are qualified to perform these services and have certifying agencies. Call the American Association of Nurse Anesthetists (AANA) at 1-847-692-7050 to determine if the doctor's recommended nurse is AANA certified.

Sleuthing references

Now that you know which credentials have more meaning, seek them out. Evaluate the doctor's medical affiliation, too. In order for doctors to be able to operate in a hospital, they usually must show evidence of proper training, experience, board certification, and expertise. While possessing hospital privileges does not guarantee the person is a good surgeon, *not* having privileges should raise some questions in your mind. Once you know the hospital, see if it has been accredited by the Joint Commission on the Accreditation of Healthcare Organizations by calling 1-708-916-5600. An appointment to a surgical staff of an accredited hospital indicates that a surgeon's capabilities and performance have been reviewed and judged acceptable by medical colleagues. Remember, you should do this research even if you plan to have your surgery performed at the doctor's office!

Don't be timid about looking into a doctor's educational background. A doctor's depth and scope of

Watch Out!
Don't be misled by the number of letters following a physician's name. For example, F.A.C.S. stands for Fellow of the American College of Surgeons, indeed a prestigious organization. But it's one where the main focus is educational. Membership doesn't guarantee that the surgeon is qualified to perform any particular cosmetic technique.

training is critical as new technologies emerge. Good surgeons continually update their knowledge and skills through continuing education courses.

Many of the better continuing education courses are sponsored by a professional group such as the American Society of Plastic and Reconstructive Surgeons. Television medical news programs have exposed the sham of certain training seminars, which may be sponsored by a manufacturer trying to push a new surgical gadget. Equally suspect are the quickie weekend courses offered by another doctor who guarantees an in-depth crash course. Even if a participant sleeps through the sessions, he'll get a certificate of learning. There are no tests to pass.

You can call the American Board of Medical Specialties at 1-800-776-2378 to verify a doctor's credentials. If the ABMS doesn't recognize the doctor as a cosmetic surgeon or qualified dermatologist, you'll need to check further.

You can check credentials yourself at your local library. *The Marquis Directory of Medical Specialists* (published by Marquis *Who's Who*) and *The Compendium of Certified Medical Specialties* (published by the ABMS) list surgeons who are certified by medical boards that are endorsed by the ABMS.

Narrowing your list

Make a preliminary list of three or four qualified candidates. Ideally, you will schedule face-to-face consultations with at least two doctors before making your final choice. Schedule an appointment with two of the four finalists for a formal consultation, but retain all your notes. If for any reason you feel uncomfortable with any doctor, go to the next one on your list.

Bright Idea
Many current state-of-the-art techniques weren't available when today's plastic surgeons were in residency programs. If you're contemplating a newer methodology, ask how the doctor was trained and how long he's been using the new approach. Also ask if the doctor owns his own equipment—this indicates he's willing to invest in a new technology.

Unofficially...
Prestigious medical schools and eminent residency training programs are highly sought after by first-rate doctors and their availability is limited. There is a correlation between excellent credentials often belonging to equally excellent doctors.

Cosmetic consultants

Some people are simply uncomfortable sleuthing references or even asking an associate for a name. For these people, there are cosmetic surgery consultants. Again: Buyer beware! Some consultants are actually quite good and will tailor a search just for your needs. But others are representatives for a small coterie of doctors who view the consultant as a marketing tool—a public relations firm, if you will. The prospective patient, believing he or she will be exposed to a wide range of specialists who can best meet their needs, will in fact be directed to only a handful of surgeons. These consultants reap double fees from both the surgeons and you. Wendy Lewis, a consultant who has been in business for over a decade, suggests prospects follow these tips to screen out deceptive consultants, many of whom advertise in national magazines or leading newspapers:

- Check the local Better Business Bureau for complaints against the consultant.

- Ask the consultant how many doctors he or she represents. Ask how many doctors are board certified and by which board.

- Do business with a consultant who has been in business for five or more years.

- Ask if the consultant is paid or compensated in any way by the doctor. Get this confirmed in writing before you make an appointment.

You may also wish to search your library for the September 1997 issue of *Allure* magazine, which features an exposé on how cosmetic consultants often misrepresent their credentials (see Appendix C).

Just the facts

- Keep track of all the details concerning your surgery by keeping a notebook and making up a planning list.

- Careful planning, keeping an open mind, and knowing your medical history are a few of the ways you can ensure your cosmetic surgery experience is a successful one.

- Make a budget and stick to it; avoid cosmetic surgery fever.

- Ask your source *why* a particular cosmetic surgeon is being suggested.

- Understand the basics of board certification; when a doctor claims to be board certified, ask, "Which board?"

- Check your surgeon's credentials by calling the appropriate medical board or doing some research at your library.

GET THE SCOOP ON...
Maximizing your consultations: smart
questions to ask ▪ Evaluating facilities and staff
▪ Getting yourself ready for the surgery ▪
Know your anesthesia options ▪ Take control
of your healing

Essential Presurgery Steps

Chapter 4

B y now you may have three or more names of
prospective cosmetic doctors with whom you
wish to consult. In this chapter, we'll look at
ways in which you can help narrow your selection by
actively participating in each of your consultations.
Much like job interviews, it is wise to stagger your
appointments over several days, even weeks. This
will give you the necessary perspective to sort
through much of the information that could be lost
or missed if you try to do too much at one time. This
chapter also shows you what to look for in two other
critically important service areas—the physician's
support staff and the surgical facility.

It's likely you'll need a battery of presurgery tests
and will be required to answer critical questions as
you approach the surgery date. You'll learn what
helps determine the best anesthesia option and
you'll be able to figure out how to adapt your home
for the recovery period. Finally, there's a real oppor-
tunity for you to maximize your healing period with

homeopathic aids, herbal supplements, and vita-mins. You'll learn which are the best to minimize bruising, swelling, and discomfort.

Making the most of the consultation

There's a real art to conducting an effective, mean-ingful consultation with your doctor while screening for those things that matter to you. First, there are several things that tend to work against patients. Most of us are in awe of any person who slogged through medical school, endured rigorous stan-dards, and suffered through years of sleepless nights during a seemingly endless residency, thus earning the right to charge huge fees. So awestruck are we upon meeting a surgeon that we forget to ask intel-ligent questions. Then we forget to listen. We know doctors are caregivers so we become childlike and deferential. C'mon, doctor, take care of us. So if you're going to be bullied by the trappings of the medical field, it's likely you'll get the medical treat-ment you deserve. For the consultation, you must be an active participant.

Pretend, if you will, that you are *not* about to interview a surgeon. Instead, imagine that you are seeking a pro who is going to house sit your new zil-lion dollar mansion for a couple of weeks. Or per-haps you need someone to take care of your favorite, elderly, persnickety pet. And then imagine that you're engaging these services in some exotic locale, a foreign land where no one speaks your language. If your precious possessions really matter to you, you'll use sign language, stand on your head, or shake a tropical vine to get your point across, right? Okay, you will now do the same thing with the sur-geons you are about to meet.

For each question asked, you deserve a clear, complete, and easy-to-grasp answer. Don't be satisfied with a doctor's response that raises other questions in your mind. If the doctor uses a medical term you don't understand, ask for an everyday, easy-to-understand definition. And then ask for an example of this definition. Make sure you clearly understand everything the surgeon is telling you. In other words, get the medical treatment you deserve.

Things surgeons never tell you

No doctor will begin the consultation by listing all the risks inherent to your pending procedure. And you'll never hear about that tiny little metal clip that was inadvertently left inside the last patient's nose. There are things you'll need to uncover, things your surgeon may not volunteer. You must ask difficult questions in order to locate the best doctor for you. To get the inside information you'll need, here are three things you must bring to each doctor's office:

- An open mind
- A pencil or pen and a small pad for taking notes
- An effective way to describe what part of your appearance troubles you. Use as many examples and details as possible. Avoid vapid, general statements such as "I just want to look better." Use clear, specific, unmitigated terms to describe what bothers you about your appearance.

It is the surgeon's chief responsibility to carefully diagnose the root of your problem. By consulting with more than one surgeon, you'll be able to see if one solution is consistently recommended or if there are several options proposed to you. For example, you may think two procedures—an eye lift

Bright Idea
Write down a few phrases to describe what bothers you about your appearance, especially if you're considering several procedures. Put the description away and look at it a day or so later. Is your description clear? Could it be understood by the average person? If there's a chance one person may misunderstand your needs, the doctor might be that one person.

and brow lift—are required, but each doctor may recommend a single option, or something entirely different. Listen carefully to all recommendations so you can make an informed choice.

The consultation is the time for the patient and doctor to get to know each other. Your doctor's goal is to determine if your expectations are realistic (will that small, turned-up nose you want really look in balance with your face?) and how your system is likely to perform during and after surgery. As the discussion gets underway, there are several things to watch for.

Look for confidence when the doctor explains your procedure. But conviction should be coupled with realistic expectations and a great deal of flexibility. You should feel comfortable discussing your needs and any niggling doubts or worries you might have. Again, this nagging doubt can be better evaluated after leaving the surgeon's office. During the initial consultation, you should sense that you and the physician do "click" on some level. If you have major concerns or if you don't feel you're on the same wavelength, you might want to look for another doctor.

At first, it may be hard to do, but don't place too much emphasis on personality and slick details. Some doctors are smooth talkers. Others may be reserved and take a while to think at length before responding. Obviously be wary of any doctor who has a pat positive answer that guarantees total success.

Smart questions to ask

In general, you hope the discussion will flow in an informative and pleasant manner. You are seeking answers from a professional; while many doctors view their time as a premium, you should expect an in-depth discovery session. Don't get hustled out the door after fifteen minutes. In getting the answers you really need, however, you'll want to avoid a clip, impersonal interrogation. Some doctors leave the discussion of the surgery to a nurse or associate. Such a cursory approach suggests the doctor is too busy or prefers to delegate some aspects of patient care. Find another doctor.

There are several basic questions you need to ask and they can be covered at any point in the consultation. But don't leave without knowing the answers to these questions:

- Is the doctor board certified? By which board?

- If the doctor is certified in a particular area of the body, is the procedure you're considering in that area of specialty?

You'll recall from the previous chapter that a doctor's membership in a number of organizations may mislead you about qualifications.

If the surgeon claims a board membership, ask for the name and number of the certifying organization. Then find out their requirements for certification.

The doctor should ask you about your motivations and expectations and discuss how the surgery could affect you psychologically and emotionally. It's important you be honest with the doctor about your personal relationships and family stability. Someone on the brink of a divorce, for example, may be too stressed to be a good candidate. If you're having a procedure on your face, the doctor needs to evaluate your skin in its natural state; don't wear any make-up, moisturizer, or other skin-care products to the consultation.

Watch Out!
If the board that your doctor cites doesn't require a residency, beware! Residency indicates the most demanding level of medical education under the scrutiny of experienced physicians who are leaders in the field. If the doctor is not certified to operate on the area you want changed, get another surgeon.

Early on, the surgeon will ask you to describe what part of your appearance troubles you. As a dialogue begins, you'll need to progressively cover most of the following issues. Here are some smart questions to ask:

1. Is my concern legitimate?

2. What are the most common ways to address this problem?

3. Which surgical approach do you recommend to specifically address this concern?

   Why is one technique or procedure recommended over another?

   What is your area of expertise? (Remember that some doctors are simply better at certain procedures. Many top surgeons prefer the abrading technique to remove fine wrinkles rather than laser resurfacing. Lasers are newer, but they may present problems that may compromise some doctors' expertise.)

4. Exactly what is likely to happen during the operation?

5. Where will the incisions be made?

6. What are the basic steps to completing this procedure successfully? (Even if your best friend just had a face lift done by this surgeon, don't presume the technique used and the results will be the same.)

7. How often do you perform such procedures?

8. How long will the procedure take?

9. What type of anesthetic will be used and why? If general anesthesia is recommended, who will administer sedation? What side effects are associated with the suggested anesthetic?

10. Where will the operation be done? (If it will take place in the doctor's office, ask to see the surgical suite. If it is a hospital, take time to investigate the facility as suggested in Chapter 3.)

11. How much pain will I experience after the surgery?

12. What risks are associated with this procedure and how common are the complications? Have you ever had a patient experience these complications? How was the problem handled, and what negative results, if any, occurred?

13. Can I talk to any of your patients who had the same surgery? (Doctors feel an obligation to protect the privacy of their patients, but they should be able to provide some contacts and most doctors are willing to comply. Of course, you will be referred only to patients who had good results. Still, it can be helpful to speak with someone who has been through the surgery. Make sure the patients are recent candidates.)

14. How long will it be before I can go back to work or be seen in public?

15. About how long will it take before the full effects of my operation are evident?

16. How obvious might it be to others that I've had surgery?

17. About how long will the improvements likely last?

18. What, if any, complications are likely to develop after surgery?

19. Are any medical tests required before the surgery? Which ones?

20. When may surgery be scheduled?

21. How involved are you personally after the surgery? Who normally removes stitches and so on? (It's more important that a doctor sees you than whether he or she actually removes sutures. That task is often left to a nurse or assistant.)

22. What are your fees and what do they cover? What are your payment terms?

23. Will I get a written breakout of all costs?

Before leaving, ask about an important, albeit unnerving, aspect to your surgery: If results don't match your expectations, or if your body responds differently from the norm, what consideration will be given to your situation and how will the doctor address any potential dissatisfaction?

A scrupulous surgeon will perform revisions in the first year after surgery without a fee. A minor revision may be all that's needed to make a good result great. Other surgeons may opt to reduce their fees, while others make no fee adjustments for revisions. (There may be additional fees for use of the operating facility and the anesthesiologist.) But since there doesn't seem to be a set policy, discuss how your surgeon will handle this possibility. Clearly you don't want to create the expectation that you are a surgical accident waiting to happen. But do be sure you understand what remedial steps can be taken to address any concerns you have once you've clearly passed through the long term healing stage.

Now is the time to discuss how expected and *unexpected* outcomes will be handled. You need to know the worst-case scenarios, not just the best.

When to head for the door

Most cosmetic surgeons are ethical and will offer the procedure with the least risk and most potential for improvement. But as you go through several consultations, there are some warning signs that may indicate the surgeon is not qualified or at least not a match for you. As you approach each consultation, try to decipher any hidden agendas. For example, be extremely cautious if the surgeon pushes for a procedure that goes beyond your original concern.

Be wary of a doctor who suggests a more complicated, invasive way to address your concern. If there is a solid reason for this technique, be sure you fully understand the doctor's specific recommendation for taking such an approach. Some doctors actually push a certain procedure because they were recently trained in it or have invested in costly equipment. Do you suspect this is the case? Cross off any doctor who tells you there are no possible risks involved in surgery. By now you know there are risks; these should be discussed frankly. Was the consultation informative and did you find the doctor forthcoming about complications and risks? No doctor likes to talk about mishaps, but honest ones will tell you about past complications or worse-than-expected results. The only surgeons who have no complications are those who do not operate.

If the doctor shows you a scrapbook of photographs of patients (or uses computer imaging) to show you possible results and promises that you'll have the same outcome, keep looking. Be forewarned: How your own tissue will react can't be translated into a computer screen image. Finally, if there is any lack of clarity about a doctor's

Watch Out!
If the surgeon recommends surgery that is truly not related to the issues you raise, his action may be considered unethical by the American Society of Plastic and Reconstructive Surgeons. Steer clear.

Watch Out!
If you or your doctor lies in an attempt to have insurance pay for cosmetic surgery, both of you are committing insurance fraud. And if the doctor is willing to lie to an insurance company, chances are he'll probably lie to you as well.

background or which fees will be charged, this may be indicative of overall careless handling of details.

There are actions you can take to remove any remaining doubt about your candidate's credentials:

- Call the American Board of Medical Specialties (1-800-776-2378) or check your local library for either the *Directory of Medical Specialists* or the *Compendium of Certified Medical Specialists*. Be certain the doctor is listed.

- Call the hospital at which the doctor claims to have privileges to verify that she can perform the specific procedure you desire. Do this even if your surgery is to be done in the doctor's office or clinic.

For your final checklist make sure you can answer "Yes" to all of the following questions:

- Does the doctor's specialty requisite match the area to be worked on?

- Is the doctor board certified?

- Is the doctor recommended by his previous patients?

- Did the doctor recommend a preliminary physical exam? (If not, eliminate this candidate.)

- Did the doctor discuss several possible solutions or alternatives to address your situation?

- Did the doctor solicit your reaction to her recommendation?

- Were you encouraged to ask questions and speak freely?

- Were you treated with courtesy?

- Do you and the doctor have a mutual, clear understanding of what your expectations are?

- Does the surgeon routinely perform the procedure(s) you want?

If you answer "No" to any one of these questions, you should seriously consider eliminating this doctor from your list.

There is no hard-and-fast rule about how many procedures a surgeon must perform monthly or yearly to stay proficient. Ideally, though, your surgeon should have performed your operation hundreds—even thousands—of times. However, if the surgeon's experience appears limited because a procedure is rarely performed or because she is using new, state-of-the-art equipment, have you been fully advised of risks?

Finally, make sure the proposed approximate surgery date works for you and be clear about how your recovery will be handled.

Evaluating staff and operating facilities

How can you effectively evaluate the doctor's staff and operating facility? During your initial consultation, the doctor's office and personnel tell you much about how the business is managed. Expect from the facility itself, at a minimum, clean windows, clean floors, and clean furniture. The reception area need not be a dead ringer for the cover of *Architectural Digest*. In fact, pricey designer chairs and decorative touches of expensive art send the wrong signals. But so do tatty beanbag chairs and shag carpeting from the '70s. The entire office environment and each full-time employee are likely to reflect the doctor's standards. Look for telling details and simple courtesies. The reception area and nurse's station should be tidy, with no bulging papers stuffed into folders spilling from file cabinets. You should be greeted in a warm fashion and

Unofficially...
Doctors who do office-based surgery can hire anyone to assist them, although they put themselves at legal risk if the assistant is unqualified. In a hospital, only properly trained and licensed nurses and technicians may assist during surgery.

the receptionist should be polished and know who you are and why you are there.

If the doctor is running late, you should be advised on arrival. While emergencies happen in all medical fields, you should be able to tell if this particular surgeon's office runs smoothly or if it is always behind schedule. There should be an up-to-date selection of intelligent magazines and a smattering of professional journals. Use your time in the waiting room to review any biographical material provided by the receptionist. The tone of any exchange you have with the office staff is a fair barometer of how patients are cared for. If the doctor continues to run late and no one offers an explanation, that's how it will be when you need stitches removed.

Today, the majority of cosmetic procedures, nearly 80 percent, are done outside the hospital at places called outpatient facilities. Why? Doctors may emphasize convenience, privacy, and cost savings. Indeed these are valid reasons. However, in recent years, health-insurance policies no longer cover the extra costs of cosmetic surgery that previously were reimbursed, notably operating-room costs, anesthesiology, and other hospital expenses. Even if claims for cosmetic surgeons' fees were rejected, these additional costs previously were often picked up by insurance companies. Depending on where you live, hospital and anesthesiology fees now can easily triple the total expense. To accommodate this staggering increase, outpatient facilities (also called ambulatory sites) began to spring up and now they predominate.

What are the advantages of having cosmetic surgery in an ambulatory facility? Outpatient surgery tends to spare patients the high overhead costs of a hospital room and hassle of a hospital overnight stay. At outpatient sites, the office-based operating room fee more closely represents the true expenses incurred, and there is no huge overhead associated with hospitals. Some patients and surgeons claim the aesthetics in outpatient facilities are often superior to hospitals. Finally, there are usually more nurses and other support staff per patient in outpatient facilities to accommodate questions and requests. You won't have to wait hours for a painkiller. In some places, I liken the ratio to a posh cruise ship. (But beware—this luxury is reflected in the doctor's fee!)

Outpatient facilities have some drawbacks, too. Even if your doctor's surgical suite is clean and has state-of-the-art equipment, you are still at a greater risk if something goes radically wrong. For example, a heart attack during or after the simplest cosmetic procedure can be addressed instantly in the hospital by a highly skilled emergency room or cardiac unit. Determine if an experienced anesthetist will be used for your procedure and be certain you have absolute confidence in this critically important staff member.

Another drawback to outpatient facilities is the lack of regulatory control. Unless the ambulatory surgery center is affiliated with a hospital or licensed by the state, neither the center, nor the surgical assistants who work there, have to conform to anyone's standards for patient safety or care. In other words, accreditation of ambulatory surgical facilities that are separate from hospitals, including some that are identified as "licensed surgicenters," is strictly voluntary.

Still, there are ways to see if your doctor's facility is in compliance. Call the American

Association for Accreditation of Ambulatory Service Facilities (AAAASF) at 1-888-545-5222. Certain basic requirements must include the availability of instruments to monitor a patient's vital functions and the system (and medications) to treat any emergency condition that may arise. Don't rely on a receptionist or nurse saying yes. Pick up the phone and call the AAAASF to find out. This organization also has an excellent Web site (**www.AAAASF.org**) that lists accredited surgical facilities. Most state medical boards also have information that can help with your decision.

You may choose a surgeon who is on staff at a major hospital. If so, remember that any hospital, large or small, can be well staffed, efficient, and equipped with the best technology. Or the hospital can be tainted by sloppiness, greed, and a string of egregious mistakes. For the average person to determine—beyond normal scuttlebutt—the rating of a hospital is practically impossible. You can try to estimate what the bed-to-nurse ratio is by simply calling admissions. Or you can pop up to the cosmetic surgery floor and make your own observations during visiting hours. But again, the best way to get a sense of how well a hospital runs is to talk with recent patients about their experiences.

Getting ready for the surgery

Once you've decided to schedule surgery, a few other related issues can be easily addressed as you move closer to the operation date. You'll want to have a clear understanding of the type of anesthetic you'll receive; also discuss what pain remedies your surgeon suggests to help your recovery. Keep your calendar somewhat flexible, too, to accommodate medical tests and arranging for "before" photographs. Here's what you need to know.

Becoming informed about anesthesia

Surgery requires anesthetic, either general, local, or local with sedation. The type of anesthetic recommended by your doctor is determined by your individual needs, general health, and what type of procedure will be performed. Upon arrival in the operating room, you will be administered intravenous supplemental medication and connected by electrodes to instruments that monitor cardiac activity and blood pressure. This is called *monitored anesthesia care,* or *MAC.* Most cosmetic facial procedures are performed under local anesthetic with sedation. If general anesthesia is required, an anesthesiologist or anesthetist (see the following section) will be present. Prior to surgery, you are usually allowed nothing to eat or drink after midnight on the night before the operation to minimize the chance of nausea and vomiting.

Generally, anesthetics are safer and more effective than ever before. But only people skilled and specially trained in anesthesia should be responsible for your care. It's important to know who will be responsible for your anesthesia and to check out his or her credentials as carefully as you would for your surgeon. There are two kinds of qualified professionals:

- *Anesthesiologists.* These are medical doctors who have obtained board certification in anesthesiology.

- *Certified Registered Nurse Anesthetists (CRNAs).* These are advanced practice nurses with specialized graduate-level education in anesthesiology. Most are members of the American Association of Nurse Anesthetists (1-847-692-7050).

Watch Out!
Because anesthetics can remain in your body for 24 hours or longer, make sure you discuss any potential reactions with your anesthesiologists or CRNA.

You should meet with either expert prior to your surgery to discuss the type of anesthetic you'll need.

Painkillers and other prescribed medicines

It is likely you will have other prescribed medicines following surgery. Antibiotics and pain relievers are common. Since the range of possibilities is highly individualized, be certain to ask your doctor what types of medicine he will likely prescribe. Be clear as to what the prescription is for, what the side effects are, and which reactions or complications you should be aware of. Determine before the surgery how you will have the prescription filled. You don't want to wait in line at your local druggist when you're feeling bad and looking miserable. If the doctor can prescribe a generic version that is acceptable, have him specify that on the prescription sheet. Always ask your pharmacist, as well, about any side effects.

Medical tests, lab reports, and "before" photos

Typically a round of preoperative tests is done according to what's appropriate for your age, individual health considerations, and the type of procedure. It's likely you will have the usual blood work, and perhaps other routine analyses. Some doctors prefer to schedule these tests a few days before the surgery to allow time for interpretation and retesting if necessary. These medical tests can cost several hundred dollars or more, based on your own needs and the facility.

Additionally, at some point your surgeon's office will schedule photography for "before and after" photos. This is an absolutely critical step. It permits the surgeon to have an excellent, authentic likeness for your final consultation and discussion immediately before surgery. While some surgeons want professional photos, others will take them in the office at no extra charge.

Scrutinize your photographs carefully before surgery. You may not be aware of asymmetries or other defects. Have the surgeon show you where incisions are likely to be placed during surgery. This will eliminate questions later on. And you won't waste time later scrutinizing defects that you don't recall. The photos will prove they were there.

I also urge everyone to take their own photos as well. Close-up, distant, and no-makeup shots. Shoot an entire roll. Assuming all goes well, it's fun watching the changes and improvements progress over time. Take some photos the day after surgery and then every day thereafter for a week. Then take a few at two weeks, and so on.

The professional photos will be taken from several angles (breast augmentation patients raise their arms and so on) to record overall shape, tone, existing symmetry, and other individual aspects. You may be asked to squint or furrow your brow to show definition of folds and creases.

Often these photos must be paid for in advance or the photographer may not release copies on time to your surgeon. Depending on how much surgery you are having done, these sessions rarely take more than twenty minutes and cost about $50 to $200.

Lifestyle considerations

Many busy people are consummate pros about interspersing their crammed work schedules with those pesky personal maintenance routines that drive most others crazy. However, cosmetic surgery requires its own personal maintenance routine. Even if you're not a procrastinator, you'd be surprised how many things can crop up at the last minute. Since this can create unnecessary stress,

> 66
> The photos are the best way to remind yourself how you really used to look. You forget very quickly. In a couple of weeks you wonder if the doctor should have done more. But one look at the old photos reminds you how far you've come.
> —Peter Tracy, athlete
> 99

let's talk about some ways you can streamline the process.

Using hair coloring and cosmetics

If you color your hair, it is critical that you do this as close to the surgery date as your doctor permits. This is especially critical if you are having a face lift or endoscopic brow work. These incisions remain tender for many weeks and the surrounding skin cannot be subjected to chemicals and harsh treatments. If you have any other routines—massage, pedicure, and so on—do not plan to schedule them anytime soon after your surgery. Although some patients are back to a full work schedule as soon as one week after a face lift or liposuction, don't count on it. The fatigue you feel may be greater than you imagined and simple weekly routines will prove daunting. You may think that you'll feel up to getting a manicure and other treatments the week following surgery, but don't plan on it.

Women are somewhat lucky in their use of cosmetics; often simple make-up can camouflage a healthy, healing incision after a few weeks. A dusting of face powder can remove the sheen of a new scar, or a foundation with a green tinge can diminish red marks and bruising. Both men and women can get help from professionals at any of the leading department stores. However, rather than stock up on products before surgery, wait until after and see what a pro recommends to camouflage the bruising. You'll probably find that little (or no) make-up is best. Often, trying to conceal an area with heavy make-up only succeeds in drawing attention to the area. If you lead a healthy lifestyle, take care of yourself prior to surgery, exercise extreme caution during your recovery, and interpret what your doctor says

CHAPTER 4 ■ ESSENTIAL PRESURGERY STEPS

down to every last detail, then you may be surprised about how fast the telltale signs disappear.

Wearing eyeglasses or contact lenses

A face lift or eye surgery can create eye havoc. Be prepared for swelling that will close your eyes for a few days. Contact lenses cannot be worn and it may be a while before you can slip eyeglasses on. With eye surgery, a clear, oily healing ointment is applied generously, blurring your vision completely. Don't expect to do any reading, TV viewing, or quickie in-bed desk work for a week or so. Since you'll have some blurring of vision, make sure your path to the bathroom is clear.

Potential reactions and side effects

You can save yourself a major blue period and unnecessary backtracking if you try to anticipate the things that might go wrong after the surgery. Discuss with your doctor the possibility of depression that tends to follow surgery. How will you cope? Have this discussion before surgery, not the day after, when anything your doctor may suggest is likely to waft away in the fog you're experiencing.

Ask your doctor and anesthetist what reactions and side effects you may have and how best to treat them. Also talk to patients who have had the same procedure to see what they suggest. If you can't come up with names of recent patients, ask your doctor's office to make some calls to see what recommendations can be turned up. As you go through the required battery of tests, ask any of the attendants who might be able to suggest insider tips.

Preparing for a more comfortable recovery

Depending on the procedure, you'll need to take some steps to make your recovery as comfortable as possible. Plan on making these adjustments two or three days before your surgery. (If you leave it until the day before, you'll run out of time). Here are some tips that will make your recovery period easier:

- Program your phone memory and auto dial (or have a paper handy) with important phone numbers: doctor, hospital, pharmacy, family, or friends who know about your pending surgery.

- Keep anything you'll immediately need—such as water, a cup for rinsing your mouth, tissues, and lotion—close at hand.

- Your bed should be as close to the bathroom as possible. Make sure the path to the bathroom is clear.

- Use a night-light until you've adjusted and become acclimated following anesthesia.

- Many procedures require cold compresses. Keep an inexpensive, insulated, plastic foam cooler within reach of your bed. Have it loaded with ice, some water, and plenty of extra face cloths or loose bandage material, so cold compresses are always available during the first 48 hours.

- With a face lift and several other procedures, you must elevate your upper body. Be sure you have some plump pillows for propping yourself.

- Before undergoing surgery, be absolutely clear about what kind of movement and activity are permissible. For example, with breast implants, you can't reach and stretch for a while. Make sure the things you need for the first week are near the bathroom sink or on the kitchen counter. If stairs present a problem, plan to recover downstairs for the first week and move when your doctor advises it.

Lining up help

No matter what cosmetic procedure you have, you must have someone pick you up and take you home. Don't rely on just a cab driver who won't know what to do if you get dizzy. Without exception, ask a reliable contact to meet you and get you back to your comfortable surroundings. Most doctors will ask you for the name of the person who will attend to this before you undergo surgery. Your doctor will also recommend a nurse or appropriate help to assist with your recovery. Be absolutely certain that you have the help your doctor recommends. And follow your doctor's recommendations—his *protocol*—to the letter.

Approach your surgery in top shape

You can approach your surgery in terrific condition if you treat the period before the surgery almost as if it were a special training. Since you will have much to do and many last-minute errands, plan as much as you can. To keep stress at a minimum, maintain your exercise program, get plenty of rest, and eliminate fatty foods, sugary sweets, and alcohol from your diet. Hydrate your system by drinking more water than you usually do; this will also help you cleanse your elimination system. Your doctor will give you a list of common over-the-counter products that you must avoid, including aspirin and, in some cases, certain vitamins. Ask your doctor about natural or herbal remedies that might help you considerably both pre- and post-surgery.

Just the facts

- Be an active participant during each surgeon's consultation.

- Evaluate all criteria before choosing the best candidate.

- Assume responsibility for evaluating patient facilities and staff.

- Take time before the surgery to schedule medical tests and "before" photos, fill prescriptions, and take care of other details.

- Take control of your healing and adapt your surroundings to make your recovery as comfortable as possible.

Common Corrections and Anti-Aging Approaches

PART III

GET THE SCOOP ON...
How aging affects what cosmetic surgery can
and cannot do ▪ How your skin ages, decade by
decade ▪ Assessing anatomical imbalances ▪
Different strokes for different folks: What
constitutes beauty?

Understanding How We Age

One growing trend in cosmetic surgery relates to anti-aging procedures. Apart from using sun block and following a healthy diet and exercise program, many patients are now electing to have cosmetic procedures done earlier. There are a number of surgeons who feel such an approach actually helps face lifts last longer. Waiting too long to correct deep creases and finely etched wrinkles may preclude your face or body responding to the usual rejuvenation corrections.

In this chapter, as you discover how skin ages, you may be surprised to learn that most of the underlying distress is caused long before it's apparent to the eye. This will help you better understand some of the issues that drive your surgeon's recommendation. Remember, with cosmetic surgery, there are limitations. Sure, you can undergo many operations in order to gain greater results. But are you willing to make such a costly, potentially risky decision?

Besides, your face and body are already crooked! Did you realize that everyone's face, even those belonging to the most arresting screen stars and models, are not symmetrical or even? Your face—and practically everyone else's—is decidedly uneven. Clearly, the importance of anatomical symmetry—how a face or body lines up—is one of the key aesthetic goals that guide most procedures.

You'll need to learn a simple test that will quantify how off kilter your features already are. This is important since, as you heal, you'll scrutinize aspects of your anatomy as you never examined them before. If you don't appreciate your own, God-given, natural anatomical imbalance before the procedure, you're likely to erroneously blame the surgeon for tampering with your alleged perfection. This chapter will help you raise your awareness level so you can better plan your cosmetic surgery.

How do we age?

The trend in cosmetic surgery is toward minimizing early signs of aging; face lifts and body tucks are now often done in a person's early forties rather than several decades later. Why? First, the skin is healthier and more resilient, and the initial results are likely to last longer. Second, when people experience cosmetic treatment at an earlier age, they are more likely to take better care of their health and appearance. Cosmetic surgery, when combined with a healthy diet and an exercise regime, can deliver remarkable and enduring results.

I feel great, so why do I look old?

Many theories have been floated in an attempt to narrow the dynamics of aging. Despite all the research, however, a number of key questions and controversial issues still puzzle the experts. Not all the answers are in. We know, for example, that our metabolic machinery—our gears, shock absorbers, and fuel delivery system—gradually exhausts itself over time. The body eventually wears out, much like that exciting first car purchased with an early career paycheck. Some experts feel that cellular exhaustion results from the accumulation of oxidants and other unwholesome, destructive metabolic products. In other words, despite living a clean and healthy life, something within your system may simply go awry and create havoc.

Genetic or hereditary factors are also key. We can't rearrange the DNA that has been passed down by our forebears. Some experts suggest that each cell is launched with a genetically endowed, programmed message. This cellular script guides the course of aging, practically predicting the time of each cell's natural death. Another idea that is closely related suggests that genetic mutations, which are known to occur periodically during the growth and division of a cell, may also work against the total system.

Destructive lifestyle behavior, such as smoking, carrying too much weight, or excessive alcohol or drugs, also tends to stimulate aging.

Whatever the cause, the result of aging skin is very much the same: The skin becomes thin, leathery, and wrinkled, and the complexion becomes dull and ashen.

Youthful skin has three very specific attributes:

- A certain plumpness, accompanied by a moist, hydrated surface

- Smooth, resilient cushioning beneath the skin

- Regardless of race, a certain under-the-skin vibrancy that comes from good blood flow and circulation

Unofficially...
The role of our autoimmune functions have shown that some antibodies are much like double agents; without much warning, they attack and destroy the healthy organism. Outside factors— radiation, noxious chemicals, or viral infection— can trigger this reaction.

The proverbial plump, dewy, and colorful hands of an infant are an example of these traits.

Aging skin, noticeably the neck, arms, or hands, also shows a swing in melanin production—the dark pigment that determines the amount of color in the skin—which may result in uneven pigmentation. The most obvious signs of this are the brown liver spots that appear on these areas as we age.

Why facial aging is different

In addition to these general changes in skin texture, the face has its own set of aging signs. In general, the plump, youthful fat layer beneath the skin diminishes. This fat loss (along with sun damage, another cuplrit) compromises skin tone. As we grow older, tissue support is generally weakened; if there is tooth loss, the person's jaw line is reduced somewhat by bone absorption. However, certain shaped features translate well as the person ages; they can look young well into old age. Small pert noses, sparkling eyes, a natural upturned mouth with fuller lips will impart a remarkably young look to some folks. Both actors Mickey Rooney and Judy Garland easily carried an adolescent demeanor well into their adult years. But most of us, with average facial attributes, age when the following four changes transpire, typically in succession:

1. A hollow appearance in the cheeks results from absorption of fat deposits (known as the buccal fat pad).

2. A thinning of plump skin begins to spread in the temple area as well as around the upper eyelid.

3. A general sagging occurs from the effects of gravity on redundant skin.

4. The envelope of facial skin does not shrink with the skull; more sagging becomes obvious.

Any loss of teeth is often accompanied by absorption of portions of the jaw, so the skeletal structure of the middle face also shortens somewhat.

Skin wrinkles can be divided into three major groups:

1. The first group of wrinkles are what we call *contour lines,* in which the skin close to the earlobe or around the jaw becomes less firm. Ironically, contour lines are not typically caused by age but are instead *accentuated* by age.

2. The second group are *dynamic wrinkles.* Invariably, these are caused by contraction of facial muscles that are attached directly to the skin. Most are formed at right angles to the long axis where the muscle contracts or pulls.

3. The third major group of facial wrinkles are *gravity lines.* These can be exaggerated over time by significant weight gain or any stress that pulls at the attachments to the underlying facial tissue. Diabetes, cancer, Addison's disease or Cushing's disease (which stem from endocrine disorders or thyroid dysfunction), or chronic nutritional deficiencies can also accelerate aging of the skin.

The changes that come with aging

Aging skin can be traced to basic alterations in cellular structure that can be studied only in a laboratory, under the microscope. The first signs of degeneration, of course, develop long before the signs of aging are apparent on the skin's surface. Characteristic changes occur in both layers of the

> **"**
> It's true: As we age, we shrink!
> —Actor Danny DeVito
> **"**

skin: the epidermis or upper layer, and the subcutaneous layer, the layer beneath the skin.

Imagine the simple structure of a beautifully crafted couch, a valuable antique, hand-assembled centuries ago. When new, the fabric was taut, crisp, and shiny; each pillow was plump and yielding when sat upon.

Your epidermis, is much like the upholstered outer fabric layer. Over time it gradually becomes threadbare. The melanin-producing cells in the skin decrease in number, resulting in less protection against ultraviolet radiation. Like a well-worn feather cushion, resiliency and the ability to "plump" back up are diminished.

Watch Out!
Elastic fiber degeneration that supports skin tone is markedly accelerated when exposed to the sun. The water content of the dermis begins to diminish, accounting for the leathery toughness of sun-damaged aging skin.

The underlying dermis—this determines the thickness and texture of skin—undergoes more significant changes during aging. Fibrous supporting tissue in this layer—which is composed of fibers of collagen, the main structural protein of the body—thickens. Elastic fibers also gradually deteriorate, contributing to decreased elasticity. It's as if the furniture's supportive webbing and coils have lost their oomph! The couch is not sagging yet, but it's lost most of its supple, cushioning power.

When the subcutaneous fat becomes less thick during aging, its fibrous connections with underlying tissue become extended. Eventually there's loss of support. This is why skin, like that fine couch, eventually droops and sags.

The aging process, decade by decade

Although sagging and wrinkling of the facial skin vary tremendously from person to person because of both hereditary and environmental factors, they generally follow a characteristic cascade with each decade: From the forehead to the eyes to the nose and mouth to the chin and neck. Here's what happens at each age group:

- *Twenties.* The first facial wrinkles are usually horizontal furrows in the forehead. Perhaps we frown a lot making our first important choices. These first expressive creases may occur in the early twenties.

- *Thirties.* Sagging of the upper lids begins and is accompanied by the appearance of "laugh lines" or "crow's feet" around the outside corner of the eyes.

- *Forties.* The laugh lines deepen (perhaps because we're all so happy by then!), and the skin of the upper lid becomes increasingly redundant, creating a hooded appearance. A sharp line of demarcation between the lower eyelid and cheek is often apparent. The under-eye area may start to look puffy. The nasolabial folds—those lines that travel from the nose down to the outside of the mouth—become more prominent during this decade, and sagging skin over the lower jaw starts to form the jowl. "Marionette lines"—lines from the mouth that travel downward on each side—can become more apparent.

- *Fifties.* The outside corner of the eye begins to droop far greater than before, resulting in a tired or sad appearance. The nasolabial fold becomes deeper and may continue toward the chin as a deep furrow forms. The skin of the neck begins to sag, and an accumulation of fat beneath the chin may produce a double chin. Stretched neck muscles often contribute to formation of bridle-like bands that travel in a vertical direction, creating the "turkey gobbler" neck. The platysma muscles on each side of the neck relax and produce bands in the neck, part of the "turkey gobbler."

▪ *Sixties and older.* Vertical wrinkling of the lips may occur. Absorption of fat tissue in the cheeks and temples gives these areas a hollow appearance. Absorption of fat beneath the eyelids may also produce a hollow or sunken appearance. The tip of the nose may also begin to droop, producing an unattractive profile with a longer-appearing nose and shorter upper lip.

Some changes can be slowed. Facial exercises won't really do much to lift sagging features, but eliminating scowling or frowning will keep your brow smoother. How can you break such habits? Some experts suggest placing a piece of surgical tape where the crease is most obvious. This little reminder, practiced over time, can actually help you correct certain negative expressions that seem involuntary but are frequently within your control. Remember, however, that some responses do one's spirit good. Laughing and smiling rejuvenate the soul and can elevate your mood—so don't stop enjoying life just because you're afraid of getting a few wrinkles!

Evaluating facial balance

As in any cosmetic procedure, optimum results can be obtained only after careful preoperative assessment and selection of proper candidates. Not all people can receive the same benefit from a surgical face lift. To appreciate how you may benefit, let's examine the symmetry of your face.

Before considering a face lift or any anatomical change—say a nose job or breast implant—take an inventory of your overall anatomical balance. Your features may be a bit more crooked than you ever imagined. Your doctor will evaluate your features very carefully during your consultation and should discuss this and facial/body proportions as well.

One of the best ways to determine facial symmetry is to take photos of yourself and cut and paste the two left or two right sides together. Or try this simple test: Look directly in the mirror and imagine balancing a coin on your nose. Slowly raise your nose; don't drop the coin! Keep your eyes fixed on the tip, trying to catch a glimpse of the coin's underside. Hold that pose and begin to examine where facial features rest or "fall" over the face. You may notice that one eye is a bit wider than the other. Perhaps your nostrils flare in an uneven fashion. Or they flare evenly, but the whole nose veers slightly to one side. Other angles may appear less uneven, too. Ears may not line up, or one may appear larger. Your jaw's right side may not match the left, and so on. Don't panic! Everyone has facial imbalances. But this discriminating eye is what the best surgeons bring to your evaluation.

It's hard for most of us to pick out these nuances; we're more likely to notice our crooked tie or untamed cowlick.

Appreciating your body's anatomy

You can appreciate the anatomy of your body in the same way as we appreciate a beautiful painting of a landscape. You approach the work of art as your eye takes in the overall view. You may scan the sky and the tops of trees, or explore the pale blue mist of the mountain ridges before you notice a charming picnic scene in the foreground. In the same painting, if there were a raging fire or flood, it's likely your eye would be drawn to that feature first.

No two paired structures of the body are mirror images of one another. Only when the discrepancy is *significant* does the asymmetry need to be addressed.
—Dr. Paul R. Weiss, cosmetic surgeon

We evaluate the human body and face in much the same way. In profile, graceful curves of the face and body that do not startle the eye are pleasing. But a large rear end may attract our eye and detract from the person's other, more beautiful features.

In a facial profile, a receding chin makes practically any nose appear too small or too large. No nose—even the most perfect one—is given a harmonious fair shake if the chin recedes or pushes out in a distracting way. We often notice the small imperfections first, much like we notice a small dent in the fender or ding in the windshield of a beautiful new sports car.

Most cosmetic surgery depends on the favorable position of the skeleton. Clearly muscles play a significant role. But bone placement is critical; it's the foundation on which all cosmetic surgeons work.

What is beauty, anyway?

There is a great deal of subjectivity about what constitutes beauty. Early in her career, some beauty expert—perhaps a casting agent—told legendary beauty Marilyn Monroe that the space from her nose to her lip was too short! She fretted about it her whole career and was never able to feel comfortable with her so-called imperfection. This is an example of how silly beauty guidelines and anatomy measurements can be.

The head is divided into two equal parts and the overriding shape of the face is oval, like an egg. Some real-life variations on the common ideal include:

- Triangular shape (the forehead is broader than the chin which is pointed)

- Square-shaped

- Round-shaped

Unofficially...
The average person measures about seven heads—more or less—high. The typical fashion drawing, however, exaggerates the proportions, making the lithe female figure nine or ten heads high!

The face falls into three basic parts. The first third is from the hairline to the upper lids. The next third is the upper lids to the base of the nostrils. And from the nostrils down to the chin creates the remaining third segment.

Here are some of the basics which our society, for the most part, feels contribute to a person's general attractiveness. Very often a surgeon will use some of these measurements when evaluating features:

- The upper lip tends to be fuller than the lower lip. In general, narrow, thin lips are associated with aging and often are less appealing than fuller, more robust lips.

- The ideal shape of the nose is a personal preference but the focal point—the tip—is often slightly above the plane of the base of the nose when seen in profile. A desirable nasal tip is thin and somewhat delicate, forming an equilateral triangle when viewed from the base. The nostrils are equal in size and oval-shaped.

- Eyes, our most expressive facial trait, are separated by the "average" length of one eye, are symmetrical, and are devoid of sagging upper lids which may convey a sad or tired expression.

- Ears rest against the head in a generally flat manner with the base of each lobe about even with the nostril line.

- The chin, viewed sideways, creates an approximate 90 degree angle with the neck. Ideally, the chin creates facial harmony and tends to line up with an imaginary line dropped perpendicular to the border of the lower lip.

Variables by sex and age

There are differences for men and women about what constitutes attractiveness. A virile young man is often noted for a flat stomach and broad shoulders that are wider than his waist and hip areas. His back is straight and lean, as are his limbs and neck. His upper body is an inverted triangle, the pointy side facing his feet. Even from a side profile, a man carries bulk above his waist rather than in his rear end, stomach, or hips.

A healthy young woman is also lean, but a certain layer of body fat rounds her body, making her bosom, face, knees, thighs, and rear end more curvy and less angular and sharp. The upper-body triangular shape of a woman is opposite that of a man. From the profile, a woman's ample bosom is often still balanced by a rounded lower body.

It's no surprise that as we age, these distinctions become less apparent. Men develop potbellies, and women can gain upper-arm fat while the bosom—especially after childbirth—can lose its heft.

There are differences in facial features, too. In general, a receding chin may be more obvious on a man's face and less desirable. We sometimes equate a man's chin with strong character. Women's features tend to be more refined; eyebrows are delicate and so is the cupid's bow of the upper lip. Minor fat deposits under the cheeks create a softer, more feminine look. A slightly protruding brow can make a man appear rugged. On a woman, however, this trait may make the top third of the face appear too thick or heavy.

Many remarkably handsome men and beautiful women defy rigid or silly aesthetic rules that seek to define ideal beauty. Conversely, many average-looking people can achieve compelling results simply by adding a chin implant or reducing the size of the nose. And that difference allows them to become the "ideal" they wish for!

What a face lift can and cannot do

The face-lift operation is most effective in eliminating sagging, redundant skin around the jowls and upper neck. While some improvement in the deep creases extending from the base of the nose to the corner of the mouth (nasolabial) can be expected, deep creases require additional measures to satisfactorily eliminate them.

Wrinkled and sagging eyelid skin is not amenable to correction by the face lift; it requires the blepharoplasty procedure for improvement. This operation is often performed in conjunction with the face lift. Fine vertical wrinkles around the lips or other areas of the face may also require other corrective procedures, most commonly chemosurgery, dermabrasion, or, most recently, laser treatment.

The double chin and the firm bridle-like bands that may be present in the front of the neck are not corrected by the standard face-lift operation. These conditions necessitate other measures, such as chin or neck liposuction, a chin lift, chin implant, or a combination of these alternatives. Sagging or webbing of the upper neck resulting from a recessed chin cannot be modified by a face lift. Such webbing is usually hereditary and present since early adulthood.

It is important to realize that the face lift cannot improve the quality and texture of the skin. Thin, poorly hydrated, weather-beaten, or leathery skin etched with multiple fine lines cannot be effectively plumped up and rejuvenated by lifting and redraping the skin.

Moneysaver
Deeply creased nasolabial folds may not vanish with a face lift. Also, frown lines and deep creases in the forehead are not corrected by the standard face-lift operation. Rather than undergo multiple procedures, you might be able to make minor corrections with injectable collagen, which, though it must be continually repeated, can postpone certain creases from deepening and last over several years.

Bearing in mind that faces are uneven, expect that some results will also appear more uneven at first. This is normal! One cheek can look larger than the other; one eye can seem wider than the other. There may be some imbalances that are obvious before surgery and some of these may be reduced or eliminated during your operation. Be sure to discuss this possibility with your surgeon. However, do not expect that your recovery, bruising, and swelling will necessarily follow an even, symmetrical progression. Also, keep in mind that in some cases, swelling may shift all over your face the first two to three weeks after surgery. In some areas, such as under the chin, the swelling will seem puffy and rock solid. Again, don't assume the surgeon didn't lift that area to your satisfaction. More than likely, it will all soften up and then tighten to meet your expectations.

Just the facts

- Skin plays a pivotal role in cosmetic surgery.

- Understand the basics of aging so you won't expect your surgeon to perform miracles.

- Adjust your expectations when it comes to facial and body symmetry; no one has perfectly even facial features and anatomy.

- The rules of proportions—the typical guidelines for what makes a face beautiful should be applied judiciously.

- Use a great deal of flexibility when assessing what you want fixed, and be aware that there are some things cosmetic surgery cannot fix.

GET THE SCOOP ON...
Vacuuming fat and cleaning up contours with
liposuction ▪ Can you use a lift? ▪
Are implants for you? ▪ Nips and tucks ▪ Skin
resurfacing: finding the soft, smooth skin you
were born with ▪ Getting the inside "scope" on
endoscopy ▪ Flaps: a way to cover up ▪ Adding
color with cosmetic tattooing

Methodologies: The Basic Cosmetic Procedures

Chapter 6

There are several ways to travel from London to Paris. A person could fly, take a ferry, or drive the underwater EuroStar passage, popularly known as the Chunnel. Cosmetic surgery,— the varied methodologies a surgeon selects to achieve a certain aesthetic goal—can be a lot like travel. Some methodologies are more cost efficient; it's simply less expensive to have a few collagen injections than to have a full face lift. Other methodologies are extremely reliable and give the surgeon a sense of familiar comfort.

This chapter helps you plan your journey to a new image by giving you the basics about the most popular cosmetic approaches. With this information, you can better discuss your surgeon's rationale behind any recommendation made during your initial consultation. What's your ultimate aesthetic destination? Do you wish to appear slimmer? Are you anxious about recent signs of aging? Have you always been bothered by a nose that seems to invite teasing, whether real or imagined? This chapter fills you in on the varied tools and methods a surgeon might use during certain procedures.

However, don't lose sight of the journey as you become enthused about technology. There are many other variables in planning a trip—duration of the trip, what you can afford, the skill of the people who pull the entire trip together, and so on. And cosmetic surgery also has variables—general anesthesia versus local, for example. These variables are covered in greater detail in the chapters that explain the various cosmetic procedures.

Which methodology is best for you?

Aesthetic methodologies have increased dramatically; cosmetic surgery no longer offers just a few ways to "get you there." Since you're the one who is paying for the trip—and will endure "recovery layovers"—you must be highly informed about each methodology. This chapter demystifies popular methodologies and reveals the state-of-the-art developments that distinguish each approach. With so many options capable of delivering similar aesthetic results, it's to your advantage to become more involved in the methodology selection process.

For example, there are five popular means of resurfacing or smoothing the skin: chemical peels, dermabrasion, laser treatment, synthetic implants, and collagen or fat injection.

Another variable is how the number of methodologies—the techniques themselves—have been refined and streamlined. Fatty deposits in the jowls used to be removed by spooning out the surplus through a surgical opening. Today, a suction device with a small tube vacuums the fat out through a smaller incision. In some procedures, advancement reduces risks. In others, the improvements may create a different liability or present a new series of side effects. Why one methodology may be preferred over another has much to do with the patient's individual circumstance and healing ability. But that is not the only criteria. Ultimately, it all comes down to the surgeon's preference. As a result, there are many incidents of patients being treated by a technique that truly does them a disservice.

In rough approximation of their order of use by surgeons, the following methodologies—and their inherent risks—should be fully explored by any person considering these cosmetic approaches.

Liposuction

Lipoplasty, commonly known as *liposuction* or suction-assisted lipectomy (SAL), is the most popular approach. It is used to varying degrees in nearly three quarters of all cosmetic procedures. Still a fairly recent addition to the field, it was developed in France as an abortion procedure, then adapted for cosmetic use. The cosmetic procedure was introduced in the early 1980s to Americans who created such a demand that the procedure rapidly made quantum leaps in technology to provide superlative results.

Liposuction is a straightforward technique that can be applied to practically any area where contour improvements can be made by removing fat:

- Face and neck, including double chin
- Abdomen and flanks, including potbellies
- Thighs, hips, and knees

> **"**
> *Incision* is simply the cutting open of an area—skin, tissue, and so on; *excision* is the cutting out. For example, prior to liposuction, an incision is made in the skin so that the cannula tube can be inserted. Unsightly skin tags, those small imperfections that seem to sprout in middle age, can be cut out, or excised.
> —Dr. Gerald Imber, plastic surgeon
> **"**

Originally liposuction was recommended for the very young whose skin had greater elasticity to rebound. Today, however, improved technique and greater medical learning provide many middle-aged patients and older prospects with successful results. While liposuction alone can produce great results, it is often used as an adjunct to a variety of other procedures. For example, men opting for a face lift may have their chin or jowl area liposuctioned.

There is an enormous misconception about general lipoplasty: It *cannot* effectively transform an obese person into a svelte reincarnation. Liposuction is not a remedy for obesity. The best results are delivered to adults who have dieted successfully, kept the weight off, and despite their healthy lifestyle, including exercise, cannot diminish certain fat deposits. It's a popular remedy for those so-called bulging "riding britches" that appear on the outside of a woman's thighs.

There are three distinct methodologies:

- General or traditional liposuction
- Ultrasound-assisted liposuction (UAL)
- Tumescent liposuction

All share many common elements. The surgeon inserts a hollow metal tube—the cannula—through an incision. Cannulas range in size according to the area to be treated, some are slight like a mini-waterpick, 2 mm in size; larger ones can be 10 mm.

The forerunner: traditional liposuction

In traditional liposuction, the doctor makes a jabbing motion with the cannula to break up fat. Since there's no complete way to avoid tearing nerves and connective tissue, significant postoperative pain and swelling may occur. The yellow gelatinous fat and other fluids, including blood, are drawn through the tube by an external suction pump to a canister where it is eventually disposed of like all medical waste.

While each surgeon's approach is as unique as his or her fingerprints, the procedures I have observed for stomach and buttock areas were startling for their apparent rough handling. The surgeon was required to repeatedly push the cannula forward and then pull backward through the fatty tissue, breaking down the deposits and removing the fat through a tube. For some patients, lipoplasty is major surgery and the resulting trauma explains why the body subsequently can ache so profoundly. In all forms of lipoplasty, great care must be taken to remove the correct amount of fat; too great a loss can result in a rumpled or unbalanced appearance, which can be difficult to correct. Fluid loss, including blood, is minimal, except in cases of large-volume liposuction in which excessive amounts of fat are removed. Those procedures are beyond the scope of cosmetic surgery and must be performed in a hospital, with intensive postoperative management of fluid balance.

The incision typically is concealed in one of the bodies creases such as the cheek fold under the buttock. Although the changes are usually immediately apparent, final results may not be completely apparent for several months due to swelling. The treated area must be wrapped tightly in a restrictive girdle-like garment to minimize swelling.

The fat zapper: UAL

UAL is a relatively new liposuction technique that uses sound waves to transform fat into a fluid. Since there's an extra step to liquefy the fat first, UAL is

Watch Out!
There are no state or federal laws that govern the depth or merit of specialty education a physician must achieve in order to call himself a specialist in lipoplasty. Serious medical complications including shock and death are rare but can occur when excessive volumes of fat are removed.

Bright Idea
Usually, only a small amount of blood is lost through UAL but, if your surgeon determines beforehand that a blood transfusion may be required, you can donate your own blood in advance and avoid unnecessary worry.

generally a somewhat longer procedure. A special combination of salt water, local anesthetic, and adrenaline is injected into the area to be suctioned. The cannula is inserted beneath the skin and the energy emitted breaks down the walls of fat cells. As fat flows out of each cell, its liquid form combines with the injected material, creating an emulsion which is then removed from the body. Generally UAL is not a substitution for traditional liposuction; it can be, however, an effective means for removing fat from fibrous body areas. These include male breasts, the back, and below the ribcage.

Also, larger volumes of fat from one area can be accommodated. UAL requires a slightly larger cannula so the accompanying incision is larger, making it less desirable for the more visible areas such as the neck. And, depending on the extent of the procedure and your individual situation, you may need a blood transfusion (although this is unlikely).

UAL was brought to the forefront through medical literature in 1991, and several thousand patients have benefited from the procedure worldwide. Unlike traditional lipoplasty, UAL often delivers its own temporary glitch: Prospects may suffer some skin burning caused by the heat delivered by the ultrasound device.

First you swell, then you shrink: tumescent liposuction

Another technique, tumescent liposuction, can reduce postoperative bruising, swelling, and pain, giving the patient an earlier glimpse of what the final results may be. Use of this technique tends to minimize blood loss, reducing the likelihood of a transfusion. Any patient who is a candidate for traditional liposuction is also likely to be a good tumescent methodology candidate. A special anesthetic liquid is injected into the area to be treated, causing the fat pockets to become swollen or tumesced. This expanded action allows the cannula to move more smoothly beneath the skin as the fat is removed. Rare complications associated with the tumescent approach—sometimes known as the *super-wet methodology,* and quickly becoming the norm—include the collection of fluid in the lungs (which may occur if too much liquid is first administered) and toxicity from a too high content of the numbing lidocaine. As with any procedure, the skill and experience of the surgeon are critically important for superb results.

With local anesthetic, you are likely to feel some warmth and a vibrating sensation. Liquids through an IV (intravenous) tube will regulate the balance of your fluids. During the postoperative period, fluid is likely to drain from your incision.

No matter which methodology is used, for large areas, the four- to six-week postoperative time includes continually wearing a snug elastic garment to help your skin shrink to its new contour. On average, patients require a month or more to begin to feel normal. If a prospect is fairly overweight, the skin will have a greater challenge to redrape itself convincingly over the treated area.

Lipoplasty side effects include:

- General discomfort, such as aches, tenderness, and perhaps the inability to sleep comfortably at first
- Pain
- Bleeding
- Temporary numbness
- Excessive fluid buildup

Timesaver
With all liposuction operations, if you develop a cold or skin infection, the procedure may have to be postponed. Schedule around the times you may be overstressed or prone to colds.

Complications, should any occur, are most likely to include:

- Clots that block blood flow
- Excessive fluid loss
- Shock
- Infection

Unofficially...
An article appearing in an 1991 issue of *Plastic and Reconstructive Surgery* reported that one in three liposuction patients claimed a return of fat to the same site, although most indicated their total weight gain was less than fifteen pounds. Touch-ups are often necessary to remove residual areas of fat.

Like all major surgery patients, liposuction patients often feel a bit blue or depressed for several weeks. Anticipate this possible setback and work with your surgeon to develop suitable coping strategies (see Chapter 16).

Does lipoplasty come with a lifetime guarantee? There are differing opinions as to how effective and enduring results are. On a qualitative basis, I have never encountered a former patient who later had the same amount (or more) of fatty deposits reappear. Perhaps people who have endured liposuction's cost and discomfort begin to take better care of themselves. Some medical experts proffer that once the fat cells are removed, there are fewer receptacles for future weight gain. For men, however, it appears that a potbelly, their sex-specific weight gain area, is the most likely place to experience a regain of fatty deposits.

Lifts

A *lift* simply repositions parts of the anatomy that droop or sag slightly. The perceived imperfection can be due to aging or a genetic trait such as baggy eyes or hooded upper lids. In many cases, the skin begins to stretch and lose its elasticity, along with the underlying tissue. During a lift, excess skin and the underlying fat is trimmed. The remaining tissue is lifted and held with sutures. Some of the more popular anatomy regions that are served well by the lift procedure include:

- Brow
- Face and jowl
- Neck
- Lower eyelids
- Breasts
- Abdomen
- Buttocks
- Thighs

Lifts can be performed under local or general anesthetic. Depending on the procedure and the individual patient's healing abilities, scars can be well hidden. Women considering breast lifts should be aware that scarring does occur, although in many fortunate cases, these lines eventually fade. However, before entering the pale, faded phase, most scars undergo a red or scarlet phase during the natural healing process. As the scar tightens, it may darken and become temporarily raised. This darkening phase usually fades to pale within six months.

Some lift procedures are considerably less invasive than those of a few years ago. A new device, the endoscope—described later in this chapter—permits the surgeon to perform major work through a few small incisions. This replaces a procedure in which one long incision was made across the scalp from ear to ear.

Implants

Implants are prostheses, artificial replacements, that augment the shape or contour of a person's anatomy. They are common in cosmetic procedures. Implants are used frequently to enhance:

- Breasts
- Pectoral and chest muscles (men)

- Cheek area
- Chin

Time varies for each procedure; a cheek implant surgery averages less than an hour. A chin implant can take anywhere from 30 minutes to an hour. During the procedure, the surgeon selects the proper size and shape and inserts the implant into a pocket over the front of the jawbone. A small incision to create the pocket is placed inside the mouth (along the lower lip) or in the skin just under the chin area. Usually the chin is taped after surgery to keep swelling down. Sutures on the outside, if any, are removed in five to seven days. Sutures used inside the mouth will dissolve naturally within a short time.

Despite the controversy surrounding breast implants, the methodology remains in demand by American patients who, in many cases, discount or do not seriously weigh the risks. Saline breast implants do not guarantee a hazard-free, long-term success rate and can mean double jeopardy for some patients who may have a history of breast cancer.

Overall, the troubling issues that prevail include:

- Lack of implant permanence
- Future removal or replacement
- Can compromise the accurate reading of a mammogram
- Deflation
- Formation of scar tissue around the implant
- Asymmetrical placement
- A hard and unnatural feel
- Rare bleeding or infection
- A change in nipple sensitivity (numbness)

Moneysaver
Cosmetic surgery often involves extra costs—many never anticipated by the patient. In most implant procedures, for example, the cost of the implant is extra. You can save yourself the cost of financing unexpected extras by asking if your implant is covered in the surgeon's fee.

The FDA and some doctors have expressed concern that some women who have had silicone breast implants report symptoms similar to immune disorders. These can range from mild flu-like symptoms to crippling arthritislike pain. Most procedures are done on an outpatient basis, the operation averages one to two hours, and you will likely experience varying degrees of temporary soreness, swelling, bruising, and a change in nipple sensation. Scars will fade over time, in several months to a year or more.

Tucks

A *tuck* is a procedure used to tighten a weak area. Tucks can be minuscule or large in scope and are used in various lift procedures.

An abdominoplasty (tummy tuck) is an excellent example of how tightening a large area can help the body gain its original tone and shape. A tummy tuck is done through a long incision placed immediately above the pubic area. Many of the steps are common to minitucks done elsewhere on the body. In a tummy tuck, however, the incision is not insignificant—typically it extends across the lower abdomen. Through this cut, the surgeon removes all of the extra skin and fatty tissue above the abdominal muscles. The belly button remains intact but eventually is repositioned through a new opening at the end of the operation.

Once the fatty tissue is removed, the lower flap can be lifted so the muscles can be examined. In severe sagging cases, the two vertical rectus abdominus muscles may have been separated, causing an unsightly pouch. These muscles can be stitched together from the pubic bone to the rib cage. The skin flap is pulled down toward the pubic area and

Watch Out!
If you have implants, it's likely that your scheduling of future mammograms will require a special technique. And, depending on the placement and size of the implant, mammogram results may be more difficult to read.

the extra tissue is removed. The incision is then closed and dressings are applied.

Skin resurfacing

Smoothing wrinkles and eliminating a number of complexion flaws, including hard-to-eliminate, ice-pick acne scars, are now being accomplished with the latest whiz-bang improvements to several methodologies. The most common are:

- Chemical peels
- Dermabrasion
- Laser resurfacing
- Injectable fillers

All of these procedures vary widely in their benefit delivery systems and each offers the ability to improve imperfections in a completely different manner. Some offer long-lasting results; others can be quite fleeting.

With all skin resurfacing methodologies, patients need to appreciate the scope of discomfort during the postoperative period. If the resurfacing is deep and covers a large area, the area, much like a skinned knee, weeps lymph and other fluids, eventually forming a crusty top layer; itching may be significant. Once the body heals itself naturally, the crusty skin falls away. Early on, you can't touch your skin, though in some cases your surgeon may suggest that gently placing a cotton swab on the itch itself may deliver some modest relief.

Let's look at each of the skin-resurfacing procedures. The type of anesthetic, surgical facility, and other factors will vary according to the individual patient's needs.

Getting back your soft baby skin

Chemical peels remove the outer layer of skin through the application of chemicals. There are several agents being used; three of the more common include glycolic acid, trichloracetic acid (TCA), and phenol.

Earlier solutions were more aggressive and contained a higher concentration of a caustic ingredient, phenol, which burned the outer layers of skin. When the results were positive, the outer layer healed to reveal a smoother surface of new skin. But a run of pigmentation problems and scarring—even from the work of leading surgeons—have forced the medical community to scrutinize prospects on an individual basis and screen out those with questionable or uneven skin types. Many surgeons no longer use phenol for peel procedures.

Peels share a number of common reactions. A burning sensation is felt for several seconds followed by numbness. Because the upper layer is, in effect, being burned by acid, the treated area weeps lymph and other fluids, eventually crusting over as new skin forms in the place of the previous layer. The procedure is usually performed on an outpatient basis with local anesthetic. Smaller areas such as the lips and eyes can be treated in a doctor's office, but larger areas are best done during a hospital stay.

Following the application of deep phenol peels, a mask of waterproof tape prevents the solution from evaporating and also assures a more uniform action. A burning sensation is apparent almost immediately and eventually heightens to the painful point where narcotic medication provides relief. After 24 hours, the tape is removed—the patient is sedated—and the raw, exposed area is dusted completely with an antiseptic powder. The powder application is repeated several times daily until the wound heals. A bland ointment, much like

Unofficially...
A full-face phenol chemical peel may require a hospital stay, intravenous fluids, and careful monitoring, since an irregular heartbeat sometimes arises.

petroleum jelly, helps manage the crust scabs that form over the tender, burned area. When results are successful with phenol, the skin is beautifully radiant and baby-new, though practically all patients experience skin bleaching. When it succeeds, phenol results can be spectacular. When serious problems arise, the results can be disfiguring and disastrous.

Since how phenol will perform cannot be adequately predicted, the medical community now often selects two milder peels—glycolic and TCA agents.

Glycolic acid often requires a shorter recovery time and the concentration—typically 40 percent to 70 percent—can be matched to the patient's skin type, area being treated, and aesthetic needs. Usually glycolic peels, also called AHA for alpha-hydroxy acid, involve a series of treatments spread over several weeks or months. The length of time that glycolic acid remains on the skin determines the depth of the peel and must be carefully monitored. Glycolic acid is generally not dangerous to the eye, though any tears streaming down the cheeks will result in a streaked appearance. Like all skin procedures, selecting an experienced surgeon should be the highest priority (see Chapter 3). Glycolic peels are done on an outpatient basis; sedation, if any, is usually a mild local anesthetic.

TCA differs from glycolic peels in that TCA acid is neutralized by another agent, allowing the reaction to ebb on its own. Compared to phenol, TCA is a milder peel that can achieve many of the same successful results without phenol-related risks. TCA can be used across a broad range of complexion colors, including those of African-Americans and dark Latinos. One form gaining popular acceptance is the Obagi or Blue Peel. The application is a transparent cerulean blue that permits surgeons and dermatologists to see the depth of application to each area. Successful results with Obagi have created a large and loyal following, and most procedures are completed in a succession of steps over several weeks. TCA peels are done on an outpatient basis and require no sedation.

A full-face chemical peel applied to the right patient by the most qualified surgeon can yield stupendous results. However, any patient considering this option should be made aware of the high incidence of variables that deliver uneven, disappointing results.

Buffing skin smooth

Dermabrasion uses a mechanical device somewhat like a manicurist's rotating electric buffer that tackles calluses. Dermabrasion removes the outer layer of skin, which is eventually replaced by smoother, newer, more regular skin. It's usually done on an outpatient basis with local anesthetic if the treated area is small.

The methodology is employed to erase fine facial wrinkles that can be conspicuous on the aging face, especially around the upper lip area. The abraded skin looks especially tender and pink, swells after the procedure, and can resemble a severe sunburn. Usually the skin heals within a ten-day or two-week period, but the new baby-fresh skin may appear pink and delicate for several months. Final results depend on the original skin appearance, the person's individual pigment, depth of wrinkles, and healing ability. Generally, dermabrasion works best on fair skin and fine wrinkles. Candidates with olive complexions risk a final result that may be less satisfactory, with the new skin noticeably paler. All patients must seriously manage

Watch Out!
Pores tend to be more prominent with a phenol peel and less obvious with TCA peels. In all peel procedures, sun exposure must be avoided for at least six months. In fact, keeping out of the sun should become a lifestyle consideration.

their sun exposure after dermabrasion and consistently wear an effective sun block.

Pitted scars left by acne respond well to dermabrasion if the scars are surgically removed prior to treatment. These scars often extend through the upper dermis into the deeper dermis or fat tissue. Depending on the number of ice-pick scars and their proximity to each other, dermatologists who elect excision prefer to treat no more than several lesions at a time, allowing this cluster to heal over a period of up to eight weeks. Stitching too many scars that are close together can create the appearance of a gap once the sutures are removed. Chemical peeling alone is not a satisfactory option for smoothing these lesions.

Zapping imperfections with lasers

Lasers have been around since 1960 or so. But a new generation of lasers is giving the medical community innovative options for delivering aesthetic results. In most cases, laser resurfacing is a brief outpatient procedure involving local anesthetic or MAC (local anesthesia plus sedation). It can be combined with other cosmetic approaches in which the patient may undergo general anesthesia.

How do lasers work? In simplest terms, the laser delivers an intense, pulsating beam of light to achieve a controlled vaporizing or burning away of the outer skin layer.

Lasers will likely continue to generate a good deal of controversy because the technique is dramatically dependent on the skill of the surgeon. And, like lipoplasty, there is no current state or federal guidelines to identify a doctor's laser skill. Many doctors who are not trained aesthetic surgeons have viewed laser technology as a way to increase an aspect of their practice that may be dwindling. A plethora of two-day seminars offered by skilled laser surgeons attracted doctors from a wide variety of fields; many simply are not qualified as cosmetic practitioners. The variable is not which laser does the best job, it's who is holding the laser. Poor training of doctors and a general lack of aesthetic ability has led to a string of serious, well-publicized complications.

The three most troubling factors that may continue to plague laser resurfacing include:

- Lack of doctor's proficiency
- Wrong patient selection
- Inadequate patient follow-up

Rather than viewing lasers as a quick-fix remedy to wrinkles and certain other perceived skin imperfections, all prospects should fully explore every step that the procedure entails. If the results promised appear too good to be true, they probably represent unrealistic expectations. How qualified your surgeon is with laser expertise is the most serious criteria you need to evaluate.

Soft-tissue fillers that plump

Either collagen or a patient's own body fat, when injected into wrinkles and creases, helps fill out the imperfection through a plumping action. These two common injectable fillers share many common features and can be used alone or in conjunction with other procedures. To a lesser extent, a number of other filler materials are also being streamlined—there's a gelatin powder compound, Fibrel that is mixed with a patient's own blood as well as a thread-like material, Gore-Tex, that is implanted beneath the skin to add soft-tissue support.

All injectable filler results should be viewed as temporary. In some rare cases, people enjoy

Bright Idea
Lasers can remove tattoos fairly effectively, especially if the original design covers a small area. Many a former flower child has said good-bye to long-ago lost love through the miraculous zapping power of lasers.

seemingly long-term benefits. Others are disappointed that their new plumping disappears in a few weeks. The dynamics for duration are not fully understood and if your collagen results prove fleeting, it does not mean that other materials will last longer. The human factor plays a significant role in the success of injectables. Patients vary in their anatomy, healing ability, and physical reactions.

The outcome of treatment with injectables is never completely predictable. Aside from allergic reactions, there are rare reports of collagen complications that include infection, abscesses or open sores, and lumpiness.

An allergic reaction to fat is not a factor since the material is harvested from the patient's own body.

Collagen contains an anesthetic agent, so additional sedation is not necessary. However, a topical numbing agent helps very sensitive patients. When fat is used, both the donor site and recipient area are numbed with local anesthetic. If necessary, some patients request additional sedation.

All of us have collagen, which is a naturally occurring protein that provides support to various aspects of our skin, bones, and ligaments. Injectable collagen was approved by the FDA in 1981 and patented by the Collagen Corporation under the trade names Zyderm and Zyplast. Both are derived from bovine collagen and produced in various thicknesses to meet a patient's needs.

With both collagen and fat fillers, doctors recommend overcorrecting each site; this allows for absorption in the weeks immediately following the treatment. When large areas are treated, some minor bruising and swelling is likely and most prospects curtail major activity briefly.

Watch Out!
Collagen injections are not recommended for pregnant women, prospects who are allergic to beef (cultured collagen comes from cattle), patients who have autoimmune diseases, and those who are allergic to lidocaine, the anesthetic agent that is combined with the collagen.

Endoscopy

Endoscopy is a less invasive methodology in which the surgeon uses a small instrument called an endoscope. This instrument is equipped with a fiber-optic light source and a tiny video camera that allows the surgeon to view the surgical area. With endoscopic surgery, minimal incisions can be made and the trauma to the area is often significantly minimized. Bundles of nerves are less traumatized and long-term numbness is generally minimized. In forehead lifts, endoscopic procedures lessen hair loss and scalp scarring. The methodology is sometimes used for lifts of the cheeks and smile lines of the face but it does not appear to be as effective in correcting jowls. Some patients do report longer swelling, but the overall benefit is that the methodology is less invasive than traditional incisions.

Flaps

A *flap* is a methodology that minimizes some defect by permitting the surgeon to cover the area with something better. For example, male baldness can be minimized through the use of flaps. Scalp tissue with hair is stripped and moved to an area of the balding forehead, giving the appearance of more hair. In treating male baldness, flaps are often taken from an area close to the ear where hair tends to be more luxuriant.

Cosmetic tattooing

Tattooing is the careful application of pigment to certain skin areas to even skin tone or enhance certain physical attributes. In some cases, tattooing can create an illusion as when an asymmetrical nipple area is made to appear more even. Some women use the procedure to add permanent eyeliner or eyebrow definition.

Unofficially...
Since collagen requires an allergic test and a four-week waiting period, some prospects prefer fat injectables. This methodology is called *autologous fat transplantation* or *microlipoinjection*. A patient's own fat cells are extracted, usually from the abdomen, thigh, or buttock area, and then reinjected beneath the facial skin.

Just the facts

- Your aesthetic goal can likely be reached through alternative methodologies; talk with your surgeon to determine the one that's best for you.

- Determine if your surgeon is truly qualified for the procedure he or she suggests.

- Assume responsibility for any of the likely risks; are they worth it?

- Develop realistic expectations; evaluate the cost, pain, and recovery involved in a procedure, as well as the anticipated result.

- Be wary of promises of perfection.

Rejuvenating the Face

Chapter 7

I s there such a thing as a minilift? You may have read articles about it, and television has done a good job of creating buzz about exciting mini-surgeries you can schedule over your lunch hour. Imagine returning to the office as a younger person! Not so fast, dear reader. There is a consensus about many miniprocedures: mostly that you get mini-results. New York plastic surgeon Dr. Gerald Imber is very likely the country's leading practitioner of the S-lift, a modified version of the more complex facioplasty. (The "s" refers to the shape of the incision, which is made in the temple area, behind the hairline.) Dr. Imber underscores the S-lift's limitations: It's effective on patients who have only mild sagging and few wrinkles. If you have major sagging and aging, there is no such thing as a minilift. He has a philosophy that I'll paraphrase: If you come into his office with lots of wrinkles, they're part of you. He can do his best to rejuvenate your face, but there are no guarantees that every line or wrinkle can be removed or even minimized.

Well, then, what options are open to you? You can have the underlying sagging corrected through a face lift. If, however, not all the fine lines will be removed, you may wish to have areas of your skin resurfaced. I'll cover chemical peels and dermabrasion in this chapter. Maybe you just want to have a few wrinkles plumped up. The simplicity of collagen (or your own fat!) injections is also described here. You'll learn why a face lift only mildly improves an aging neck and how the neck can be redraped with a face lift. I'll cover the major procedures for rejuvenating the face in this chapter, including how much each procedure costs on average, how long each procedure takes, possible types of anesthesia, and other pertinent details. Do you want one procedure done or possibly a combination of several? I'll explain how you can save time and money by combining several procedures.

Face lifts: making the face look naturally refreshed and younger

One of the more interesting variables about face lifts, forehead lifts, and eye jobs is that you really should experience no remarkable pain. No, you won't necessarily breeze through most of these procedures, though many patients do. In general, prepare yourself for general discomfort and bruising. If you beat these odds, all the better. Expect peculiar swelling, some pain, or an uncomfortable sensation of tightness, even numbness, around the suture areas and elsewhere. Each procedure offers its own set of potential reactions. Exactly which procedure is recommended typically is based on several variables, including:

▪ Surgeon's preference and expertise

- Your appearance
- Your health and medical history

The following surgeries and matching summaries provide basic details. Many individuals can look much improved with only a simple eyelid operation; it takes a few hours and can be done on an outpatient basis. Your surgeon may recommend a combination of several procedures for optimal benefits. In addition to an eye job, excessive facial skin and a slightly jowly chin can be improved only by face-lift surgery. (Excessive neck sagging requires a separate procedure, which I'll cover in Chapter 9.)

Bear in mind that the following prices represent a national sampling. Usually, all other fees, including operating room, anesthesia, medical tests, before and after photography, and prescriptions, are extra.

Common name: face lift (facioplasty)
What it does: Eliminates mild or major sagging, modifies nose to mouth smile lines, generally improves the tone of the lower face
Price range: $3,500 to $15,000
Operation duration: Three to six hours
Anesthetic: Usually local with sedation (MAC), although many doctors prefer general anesthetic if they are doing supplemental surgeries
The procedure:
The incisions for face-lift surgery are commonly placed in the hairline, in front of the ear, under the chin, and in other areas where the scars can be expected to heal very well and where they are less conspicuous. Face-lift incisions often leave no obvious scars or marks. The facial area is cleaned with antiseptic solution and sterile cloths, and other

surgical drapes are placed around the face to prevent contamination. The incision lines are then
carefully outlined on the face with a marking pen;
your before photos may be used for reference.

The usual face-lift incision begins in the natural
crease at the junction of the ear and face. At the ear
lobe, the incision continues around the back of the
ear, ascending in the crease between the ear and the
area behind the ear, called the *mastoid*. At the top of
the ear, the incision curves backward into the hairline. For some patients the incision extends into the
temple hair above the ear, generally curving slightly
forward. The surgeon may adjust this basic incision
depending on each individual patient's needs.

The following before and after photos show how
facioplasty incisions seek to camouflage scars while
permitting surgeons flexibility to manipulate the
underlying tissue. Some ear area incisions go
behind the earlobe extending up behind the ear to
the center muscle, and then diagonally back into
the scalp behind the ear.

After the incision is made in the temple area, a
dissection follows just beneath the skin and skin fat,
continuing to the fold between the lip and the
cheek, and to the midline of the neck. This is where
the surgeon separates tissue and works carefully to
avoid nerve damage. Great care must be taken or
there could be permanent loss of sensation to the
ears and to muscles that animate the face. The facial
skin is lifted and bleeding is brought under control.

The thin fascia or connecting tissue of the superficial muscle system is pulled backward in order to
provide deeper support to facial tissue, particularly
around the jaw. This tissue is then sutured to the tissue just under the skin behind the ear. Any fat on

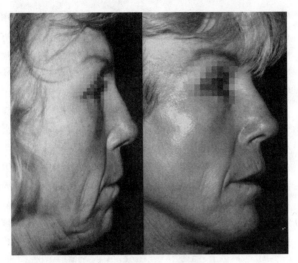

This before and after comparison shows excellent results. A small chin implant balances the final results.
(Source: Dr. Stephen Grifka)

top of that area is removed to give a sleek, clean look. Then, six to eight sutures are placed down either side of the inside neck to secure the connective tissue and muscular layer before the skin is redraped. This creates the appearance of better facial tone. A considerable amount of time is then given to coagulate all of the blood vessels. Any bleeding in the face may cause problems and potentially compromise results. The extra skin is carefully trimmed to eliminate pulling and wrinkling. The cheek skin is also pulled. Stitching is done with care in order to minimize scarring.

At the conclusion, small tube drains may be placed in the neck area (behind or near the ear) in order to siphon any oozing. A sterile dressing is applied and a helmet of bandages secures the head and neck area. Cold compresses must be applied

Unofficially...
Undermining is a surgical term referring to the lifting of one layer of tissue from an underlying layer of bone or tissue. In a face lift, the cheek area is undermined.

vigilantly for the first 24 hours to minimize swelling and bruising. The drains are removed the following day. The sutures that pull the most (or carry the stress of the new lift) are behind the ear. When healing has run its course over several months, you should have a natural, rested appearance, not a tight, masklike pull from the jaw to ear areas.

Postoperative expectations:

The average patient experiences varying degrees of pain and discomfort. However, there should be little, if any, sharp or intensely throbbing pain; many of the nerves, having been cut, are unable to deliver painful sensation. These nerve endings should successfully regenerate over time. A sensation of pressure or an almost unbearable tightness is common, but adjustment is rapid—within several days—for most people. And just when you get used to it, it's gone. Mild pain-relieving medications are given as necessary; these can range from over-the-counter remedies such as Tylenol to prescriptions such as Hydrocodone. If they don't relieve the discomfort, alert your surgeon. In general, you should keep as quiet as possible with your head elevated and limit your physical activity. No sex is permitted for at least a week to keep your blood pressure normal.

When you get up to urinate, don't be alarmed. As you begin to move a bit, you'll realize you can't really swivel your head to see who's coming into the room. This will mostly disappear within a few days and eventually fade completely within a week or so. Most bruising goes through a predictable pattern of varying colors: red and blue bruises that may brown or turn jaundiced yellow before fading. The amount of bruising varies with each individual and is impossible to accurately forecast. Unbelievably, some

Bright Idea
Place a disposable, absorbent pad behind your head to soak up the oozing from any plugs; have extra pillows stacked to keep you upright and cradle your head. Make sure you have someone to help you rotate cold compresses.

patients look almost normal within a few days. Some patients go right into the final yellow stage, with just dabs of light bruising and slight swelling; others have a more dramatic appearance, with black-thread sutures, swelling, and significant bruising.

A liquid or soft diet is usually prescribed for 48 hours to avoid use of chewing muscles. Before the first dressing is removed the following day, be warned that the face may appear swollen and discolored. Or it may simply appear puffy, pulled tight with no bruising. The hair is usually matted and, having been swabbed in antiseptic, it's going to feel sticky, as if dipped into a barrel of hair gel. Some surgeons approve of careful shampooing with a mild shampoo two days after the procedure, others may want you to wait longer. The sutures in front of the ear are removed on the fifth postoperative day. Those behind the earlobe and up into the hairline—temporal and mastoid sutures—are taken out near the seventh or tenth day. (The sutures at the two points of maximal tension, shown in the previous photo, are removed 14 days after surgery.)

You are normally checked again a week later and then again four to six weeks after surgery. Of course, if you have *any* concerns about even the smallest pain or unusual swelling, call your doctor that same day. And first-week to ten-day swelling, though normal, can be startling; some little pockets may resemble a smallish hard-boiled egg on the nape area or behind the ear. Some areas may have to be drained; others subside on their own. Let your surgeon see what you consider to be a problem. If it's a real issue, the doctor will treat it appropriately. If it is just part of the normal healing process, at least you'll get reassurance and be able to relax again.

Timesaver
Staff nurses routinely remove stitches; most are usually extremely skilled at this. Don't worry about allowing them to do their job; your surgeon can check you afterward.

Gradual resumption of simple activities is recommended; walking will help galvanize the healing process. But do not bend over for three weeks or more. If you must bend, stoop at the knees, keeping your head upright. Never lift anything heavy or strenuously place pressure on the sutures. Vigorous activity should be avoided for one month—no weight-bearing machines at the gym—as they can temporarily elevate the blood pressure and result in hemorrhage under the facial skin. Your surgeon will tell you when you can resume your normal athletic routine and what you can do. Many patients return to work within two weeks. Remember: The healing process will continue internally for several more months. The best, fully realized results may not be apparent for several months or a year. After two weeks, however, you'll see improvement nearly every day until the face normalizes.

The face is usually numb in some areas because of inescapable injury to small nerve fibers that supply the skin. Regeneration of these fibers begins immediately and may be complete in six to twelve weeks, though numbness in varying degrees may continue for up to nine months or a year when final results can be assessed.

Another variation of the face lift, the endoscopic lift, is discussed next. In some areas, when this procedure is used before the age of 40 to address minor signs of aging, it is sometimes called a minilift. (Another procedure, notably the new chin lipo/laser lift covered in Chapter 9, is known as the weekend lift.)

Common name: face lift (endoscopic facioplasty)
What it does: Reduces lower facial sagging and signs of age

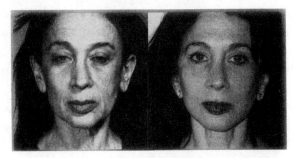

Lower facial sagging and aging can be dramatically minimized, as these typical before and after photographs indicate. Through redraping, minor neck improvement can be addressed as well, though significant neck aging requires its own remedial procedure. (Source: Dr. Gregory LaTrenta)

Price range: $7,000 and up
Operation duration: Three to four hours
Anesthetic: General
The procedure:

The endoscope is a telescope-like instrument that gives the plastic surgeon a window through which to see the anatomy and accomplish many facial cosmetic surgical procedures. A fiberoptic light source and video camera are placed through a small incision; the image is then transmitted from the endoscope to a television monitor. While watching the monitor, the surgeon is able to extensively undermine the sagging area, suture, staple, and rearrange tissue; the resulting scars are much smaller than the scars from traditional facioplasty.

An endoscopic face lift usually takes three to four hours; the surgical team includes your doctor, the anesthesiologist, surgical nurses, and perhaps a nurse technician.

Endoscopic face-lift procedures are usually accomplished in two very different ways: the superficial approach and the deeper lift approach.

In the first approach, also called the subcutaneous technique, the skin, elevated through incisions at the hairline level, is pulled and pleated. At the hairline level above or behind the ear, the pleats slowly disappear over a period of several weeks. Because no tissue is undermined after the incisions, it is known as the minilift. Typically, the overall change is "mini" as well.

The second approach lifts the deep structure of the face by freeing up the overall original attachment and re-anchoring it in a more toned state to the facial bones. The tissue and muscle are then secured at a higher, pulled-back position. Because the end result of an endoscopic lift may be considerably less than that of the traditional face-lift procedure, patients with much saggy or droopy skin, especially in the neck region, may be best served by a traditional face lift.

Postoperative expectations:

Most of the healing is less uncomfortable (and often the recovery period is shorter) than a traditional face lift due to the smaller incisions and microscopic handling. The overall general recovery is rarely very painful; since the area is less traumatized, the patient may exhibit less bruising and swelling.

Possible complications (both traditional and endoscopic):

Significant problems relating to traditional and endoscopic face lifts are infrequent and the convalescence of most patients is uneventful. The most common complication is bleeding beneath the undermined facial skin; a localized collection of blood in about five percent of cases occurs. Most blood poolings are small and resolve spontaneously without consequence. Others are large enough to have the area aspirated with a large needle.

Surgically removing too much skin can cause
tightly sutured wounds to place excessive tension on
the undermined skin. This can eventually widen the
incision and result in an abnormally wide scar. Your
doctor can probably revise this scar at a later date. A
serious complication can be the permanent loss of
sensation along the cheek area. Patches of hair may
be lost from the temporal area due to excessive tension on the facial skin or if hair follicles are injured
during the undermining process.

Skin resurfacing for a smoother you

The chemical peel—a form of chemosurgery—is a
valuable technique for rejuvenating the aging face.
Candidates must be chosen carefully! Multiple fine
wrinkles respond fairly well; these wrinkles typically
are not remedied by a face-lift operation. The chemical peel, on the other hand, does not improve the
general sagging of the skin of the face and neck. So,
in many cases, both face lift and chemical peel are
complementary procedures.

A plethora of print and TV ads, beauty spa
claims, and treatments offered by both dermatologists and surgeons, have confused many prospects
about what constitutes a peel. Here's what you need
to know: By the late 1980s, the concentration of the
original ingredient of the controversial deep surgical peel, *phenol*, had been reduced. Earlier versions
caused scarring in some cases. It is now available in
several strengths. Since then, however, more products with varied names and a range of claims have
multiplied. A peel using trichloracetic acid—called
TCA—is less invasive and works on darker complexions. (A well-known example of TCA is the Obagi
Blue Peel, developed by a California dermatologist.
Administered by a medical doctor, the peel's blue

Watch Out!
Most minor
hematomas form
in the first few
postoperative
days. However, a
hemorrhage can
occur later if you
increase blood
pressure by lift-
ing, bending
over, straining, or
some other vigor-
ous exertion.
Seriously bump-
ing your head
or disturbing
healing skin
can also create
complications.

color permits a more even application and precise depth control.) *Glycolic* peels are the mildest versions; they are stronger, however, than the very mellow fruit or natural peels, called alpha-hydroxy acid (AHA) peels, offered by spas and beauty salons.

AHA, often derived from fruit, milk, and other natural sources, is an exfoliant that speeds up the shedding of superficial skin cells. Used regularly over time, AHA products can leave the complexion with a smoother, fresher appearance. These popular beauty counter products—mild skin lotions and creams—contain a level of 10 percent AHA or less. They are considerably less potent than AHA medical remedies, dispensed only by doctors, which feature an AHA concentration of 30 to 70 percent.

Here are the different chemical peel actions:

- Phenol, the strongest chemical peel, is carbolic acid and removes the entire epidermis, down to the middle dermis.

- TCA burns off the entire epidermis and only the most superficial portion of the dermis.

- Glycolic acid, the mildest of the three peeling agents, removes only the outer layers of the epidermis.

The ingredient of each substance produces a burn of the skin. With phenol, several other ingredients are added to promote even dispersion and penetration of phenol. Most peels, except full-face deep peels, are typically done on an outpatient basis. Chemical peeling almost always causes a permanent decrease in skin pigmentation, which is more noticeable in darker skins; the line between treated and untreated skin is often clearly evident, though TCA peels have reduced this considerably.

The postoperative course of a *deep* chemical peel is perhaps more taxing than that of other cosmetic procedures, and the surgeon must be sure that the patient has enough emotional strength to weather it. Chemical peel candidates must understand the importance of keeping out of direct sunlight for three to six months. Also, since melanin production is permanently diminished by the peel, prospects may never again be able to obtain a dark tan. If a *deep* chemical peel is not an adjunct procedure—but becomes the primary surgery of the entire face—it must be performed in the hospital because of the discomfort frequently experienced during the post-operative period and the absolute need for crucial vigilance by the surgeon.

Unofficially...
Apart from complexion color, the texture of the skin is an important factor in selection of peel patients. The ideal candidate has relatively thin, moist skin. People with thick, oily skin are more apt to develop unsightly color "blips" after this procedure.

Common name: face peel (chemosurgery)

What it does: Chemically burns the skin, minimizing superficial wrinkles, brown age spots, and other minor external signs of sun damage and aging

Price range: $300 to $5,000, depending on the area to be peeled and the type of peel

Operation duration: An hour (or less) to several hours

Anesthetic: Local with sedation or general, depending on depth and type of peel

The procedure:

The patient is instructed to wash his or her face with an antibacterial soap for several days before the procedure. Some patients, depending on the depth of the peel, may also be given other topical prescription treatments, perhaps Retin-A to begin preliminary exfoliation. At the hospital, preoperative sedation is administered for a deep peel several hours before the procedure and an intravenous infusion is started through which additional sedation can be delivered as required.

Before the strong chemical solution is applied, the face is carefully washed with surgical antiseptic and ether to remove all traces of oily material. As the chemical is applied, the skin is gently stretched during application so that the solution will uniformly coat the skin and the bottom of each fine wrinkle. Application continues into the hairline and eyebrows and up to (but not on) the red line of the lips. The application is continued to a point just below the border of the jaw. The neck skin is generally not peeled using phenol because a high incidence of scarring and abnormal pigmentation are common. A very light solution, if any, is applied to eyelids since the skin is exceedingly thin and delicate.

With deep and medium peels, a burning sensation follows several seconds after each application. (When a phenol solution is applied, a mask of waterproof tape may be applied later to the skin. This mask prevents the phenol solution from evaporating and thus enhances its effect, producing a deeper and more uniform peel.)

Application of a medium or light peel differs completely. In most cases, the doctor will advise the patient how to treat the skin for several weeks or days prior to the peel. Topical applications may include a special soap or exfoliating products. The peel itself is usually performed in the doctor's office and the patient, ambulatory afterwards, returns home and stays indoors to allow the crusting stage to begin. With very light peels, many patients appear normal, though pinkish, several days to a week later. However, almost all patients prefer to wait for the scabbing and flaky crusting to disappear before facing the real world.

Postoperative expectations (deep phenol peel):
Approximately one-half hour after the deep peel is completed, the patient begins to experience a burning sensation that gradually increases in intensity. Over the next 48 hours this pain frequently requires narcotics for relief; this is a major reason for performing the procedure in a hospital. The patient rests in bed with the head elevated.

Iced compresses may be helpful in reducing paid during the first 24 hours.

On the second post-peel day, the tape mask is carefully removed and the raw area is covered with an antiseptic powder. The patient is heavily sedated at this time. The patient is usually discharged with instructions to apply the powder three times a day. Physical activity that creates even mild perspiration while the face is powdered is off-limits.

Following a deep phenol peel, the appearance—in spite of the surgeon's preoperative warnings—can be absolutely appalling. Be prepared: You will look like Lon Chaney in *Return of the Mummy*. Application of bland ointment is begun 24 to 48 hours after the mask is removed in order to promote a breakup of the crust of powder from the face. Thereafter, gentle washing of the face with bland soap and water is started to hasten crust separation. Itching can be fierce, but the face can't be touched (except by placing a cotton swab on the itch). Small blisters on the lips will disappear without any special treatment.

Postoperative expectations (medium to light peels):
Pin-sized whiteheads called *milia* frequently occur (usually around the mouth) after medium chemical peels. These areas are caused by temporary obstruction of small glands of the facial skin and, in most

Bright Idea
Chewing causes discomfort and loosens the tape mask, so to perk your spirits after your deep peel, have some healthy fruit drinks or liquid diets ready. Sipping through a straw is comfortable and the liquids will rehydrate you.

cases, can be satisfactorily treated by gentle washing. Some milia must be opened with a sharp needle.

Depending on the depth of the peel, the newly regenerating skin appears thin and delicate, and either very red or very pink. With all peels, except very mild glycolic solutions, a significant scaly crust forms and falls off, though afterward no treatment is necessary other than frequent gentle washing and application of the bland ointment to help retain skin moisture. With deep and medium peels, ointments containing cortisonelike agents are sometimes prescribed.

The following photos show before and after peel results.

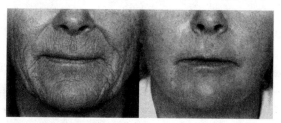

Before and after anti-aging results of a medium peel. (Source: Dr. Zein E. Obagi)

With very light peels, often procedures are done as a series, perhaps three or four sessions, extended over several weeks or months. Cosmetics may usually be applied two weeks after the peel and can diminish the red appearance. All exposure to the sun must be carefully avoided for three to six months and avoiding the sun altogether may prevent continual, excessive wrinkling.

Possible complications (all peels):

Problems that can range from minor to severe usually relate to uneven skin pigmentation results. In some cases, this is due to the unpredictability of certain skin types and may be beyond the direct control of the surgeon. Some patients develop a noticeable line of demarcation at the junction of untreated skin just below the jaw. This possibility must be carefully discussed with your doctor before you agree to the procedure. If the line is objectionable, proper use of cosmetics can help conceal it, but only you can decide if you want to assume a daily, albeit permanent, beauty routine.

Occasionally, areas of splotchy hyperpigmentation develop after a chemical peel. Again, this problem occurs most frequently in people with dark complexions, but may also occur in light-skinned patients after sun exposure. Repeeling of the face is often necessary to correct this, but it may have to be delayed long after the first peel. Pigmented facial blemishes present before the peel are frequently relatively darker after the procedure. This darkening tends to be unavoidable, so the only preventive measure is to remove the blemishes before a chemical peel. Finally, in general, skin pores appear to be more prominent.

As a postscript: Full-face peels that also accompany a face lift may be delayed for several weeks; the taut skin can cause excessive or uneven depth of the peel to occur if these procedures are performed simultaneously. However, chemical peel of the upper lip is commonly performed at the time of the face-lift operation.

Common name: dermabrasion

What it does: Removes fine wrinkles

Price range: $300 to $3,000, depending on area treated

Operation duration: Varies, depending on area treated

Unofficially...
Did you know
that removing
fine lines by
dermabrasion
remains one of
the preferred pro-
cedures of many
seasoned, top
plastic surgeons?
These surgeons
maintain that
penetration to
the precise depth
required by deli-
cate lines can be
better controlled
with dermabra-
sion. This depth
is often overesti-
mated by less
practiced sur-
geons using
a laser.

Anesthetic: Usually local

The procedure:

Dermabrasion is usually performed on an out-patient basis in the surgeon's office, but is occasionally performed under general anesthesia in a hospital operating room.

After the skin is carefully cleansed with an antiseptic solution, the area to be treated is anesthetized. Anesthesia can be obtained by injection or by freezing the skin with a refrigerant. In addition to inducing anesthesia, freezing also makes the skin firmer, helping the surgeon deliver a uniform abrasion. Deeply etched or wrinkled areas are marked with dye to help the surgeon match the proper level of abrasion to the surrounding skin. If a large area is to be treated, dermabrasion is performed in small units to ensure a uniform skin removal. The tool is a small, hand-held instrument, much like an electric callus remover used in pedicures. The abrading disk rotates at high speeds. Bleeding is controlled by pressure, and an occlusive gauze dressing applied.

Dermabrasion results can be dramatic, as seen in the following photos.

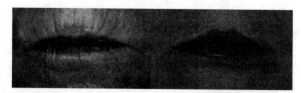

Dermabrasion can significantly reduce fine wrinkles, as these before and after photos show. Upper lip augmentation, using collagen, followed dermabrasion for a fuller, more youthful result.

Postoperative expectations:

As the gauze begins to spontaneously separate within three to five days, the patient is instructed to cover the healing area with ointment. The healing area appears intensely red, resembling a sunburn, and can become crusty and flaky. This resolves over a period of time that varies from patient to patient. In some cases a tender redness is prolonged over several months, particularly if the patient exposes herself to the sun. In other cases, the patient appears normal within several weeks to a month, depending on how deep the abrasion is and the nature of her complexion.

Possible complications:

Dermabrasion scarring is uncommon but may occur if abrasion has been too deep. In rare cases, an infection can form but can usually be easily treated with a topical antibiotic. Since certain areas such as the neck are prone to scarring, dermabrasion is not performed in these areas.

Common name: wrinkle filler (injectable collagen)

What it does: Plumps fine lines and makes wrinkles appear less deep

Price range: $300 to $1,000, depending on area

Operation duration: Under an hour

Anesthetic: Usually none

The procedure:

Collagen injection (Zyderm) is a reasonably easy, albeit short-term way to deal with fine wrinkles. Most of the lower layers of the skin consist of a large protein molecule called collagen. This dissipates as we age. To supplement yours, collagen from cattle skin is purified and made into a liquid to be injected with a syringe into fine wrinkles. It appears to be successful in most cases, but the patient must first receive a test dose to assure there is no allergic reaction. Several weeks later, the collagen treatments can be started. Collagen injections are minor procedures commonly done in an office setting, using a syringe with a very small needle. The patient's fat, instead of collagen, can also be harvested and used to minimize areas of wrinkling and depression. To do this, the surgeon liposuctions fat or uses a syringe to withdraw fat from the lower abdomen or buttocks, the most popular sources. While fat injections don't produce an allergic reaction, their results are as limited as collagen: only short-term. The procedure is performed in an office, and the patient is completely ambulatory afterward. To obtain optimum results, most doctors allow for a 10 percent overcorrection, which dissipates to normal within 24 to 48 hours.

Postoperative expectations:

Each injection tends to produce the immediate appearance of overcorrecting: The area puffs up and will subside in a few days, leaving a more normal appearance. Remember, the results are not permanent because the body gradually absorbs the collagen. Some results last only a month. Others can last longer, with six months the average.

Possible complications:

Typically there are no significant complications. However, you should always be sure that a qualified doctor does the injection. Delegating this step to an assistant or nurse could result in overcorrection, possible temporary blistering, or the needle hitting a blood vessel.

Common name: laser resurfacing (ultrapulsed laser)

What it does: Vaporizes the top skin layers and tightens underlying collagen tissue

Price range: $1,500 to $3,000 partial face; $3,000 to $7,000 full face

Operation duration: Partial treatment, up to an hour; full face, less than two hours

Anesthetic: Local, though many surgeons prefer general anesthesia for a full-face procedure

The procedure:

Ultrapulsed laser is the short name for the pulsed carbon-dioxide (CO_2) laser beam. Around 1992, this new technology created an industry buzz because one important difference was perceptively superior to older lasers: less chance of skin burn, called charring.

The new laser deftly delivers minibursts of light. So, like quickly passing a finger through a flame, the skin doesn't get scorched. A pulsed laser vaporizes the top layers of skin and tightens the underlying collagen tissue. When the new skin grows back, wrinkles, skin tags, and other signs of aging are reduced or, in many cases, eliminated. The laser works much like a peel in that the top layers are destroyed, literally vaporized, as the following before and after photos indicate.

Unofficially...
Traditional lasers deliver a continuous beam of concentrated light energy and almost always fail in cosmetic surgery because they char the skin.

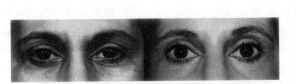

Eye areas often respond well to laser resurfacing, as these before and after photos show. (Source: Dr. Gregory LaTrenta)

Your face is cleansed with acetone to remove facial oils and is marked with a surgical pen to delineate the area to be treated. An antibiotic solution, usually Betadine, is applied to kill topical bacteria. To prevent penetrating too deeply, the laser can be programmed. The pulse rate can range from 10 bursts a second to more than 500 bursts a second. The shorter the burst, the lower the energy, and the less penetration. The most sophisticated lasers have robotics that increase accuracy. The surgeon makes several passes over a small area and, usually, by the third pass, the underlayer is exposed and the laser beam shrinks the collagen. The procedure is bloodless since the heat instantly cauterizes blood vessels. If you are awake, you will hear the crackle of zapping, smell a bit of smoke, and have a sensation much like someone snapping a tiny rubber band against the skin. (A vacuuming tube minimizes vapors.) If your mouth area is being treated, your eyes are covered by a surgical drape or other protective gear. If your eyes are being treated, anesthetic drops are put in your eyes, which must also be protected by a steel lens.

Postoperative expectations:

The skin will appear raw and red. A clear ooze, much like the lymph that accompanies ruptured acne, will make the face appear wet and shiny. Any redness, which is often significant, may take up to 14 days, perhaps longer, to fade. Much of this will depend on how much surface was treated, the expertise of your surgeon, and your own healing capability.

In some cases, bandages are required. Some surgeons apply Flexzan, a biomembrane tape, which retains moisture and reduces pain while it speeds healing. The tape stays in place for seven to ten days during which time it must remain completely dry. You will have to bathe rather than shower and someone will have to wash your hair. Enduring the bandage treatment, however, usually gets you back to normal in a speedier fashion. Without a dressing, pain and discomfort can be managed with an over-the-counter painkiller. Your face must be washed four or more times a day. Crusting must be dissolved with peroxide and, after each cleansing, your face must be coated with an ointment such as petroleum jelly.

Be aware that since the skin is swollen at this time, you may think your results are completely wrinkle free. As soon as this puffiness subsides, some wrinkles will begin to appear.

Possible complications:

As with other cosmetic procedures, infection is a risk, both bacterial and viral. Any history of shingles or herpes must be treated before the surgery with anti-viral drugs. If the skin is vaporized too quickly, or the peel is delivered by a surgeon with little expertise, scarring is a significant possibility.

Additionally, a number of cases where the lower eyelid was pulled, forming an ectropion (which I'll discuss in the next section), have been reported. This is attributable to the collagen under the skin tightening excessively. Laser surgery is not to be taken lightly; the doctor must have rigorous training and expertise. If the laser beam hits an unprotected eye, blindness can result. Finally, because the procedure is so new, there are no long-term studies on how long improvements may last.

Common name: eye job (blepharoplasty)

What it does: Restores a refreshed, more youthful appearance to lids; removes tired lines, bags, and general puffiness

Price range: $1,500 to $7,000, depending on whether single or upper and lower lids are done

Moneysaver
Your skin surface must not dry out, and vigilant moisturizing is part of the strict regimen. Many patients recommend Crisco—it's inexpensive, slathers on gently, and seals the skin. And a small supply will last your whole recovery period!

Watch Out!
Before and after photos of laser resurfacing can mislead you if the *after* photo was taken when the area still experienced some swelling, thereby reducing signs of wrinkles.

Operation duration: Single-lid procedures average an hour; both lids average three hours or less

Anesthetic: Usually local

The procedure:

The eyelids are among the first areas of the face to exhibit signs of aging—perhaps 10 years before other facial areas begin to age. Eye aging begins with the development of crow's feet at the outer corners of the eyes during the late twenties or early thirties. Next, sagging of the skin of the upper lid begins and produces hooding that is especially marked in its outer half. Fat resting in compartments between the skin and muscle of the lower lids may protrude, producing pouches or bags that result in a tired or sad look. Sagging of the outer corner of the eyelid and eyebrows reinforces this impression. An effective eye job—many are first done in the late thirties or early forties—can significantly rejuvenate the face. For many prospects, at the right time and done well, an eye job can give a much younger appearance, erasing the past 10 years or so.

The eyelid skin is thin and delicate. A characteristic furrow, the *superior palpebral fold,* is present in the upper lid when the eye is open. Beneath the eyelid skin is a muscle, which surrounds the eye in a circular fashion and is responsible for closing the eyelids as well as aiding the flow of tears. Contraction of this muscle (even squinting) causes crow's feet and, as we age, the aging eye appears less wide, adding to the illusion of fatigue or sadness.

The blepharoplasty consists of removal of excess skin, muscle, and fat from around the eyelid.

The facial skin is cleaned with an antiseptic solution and sterile surgical material is draped around

Moneysaver
Many patients elect to have only upper or lower lid surgery. The cost efficiencies for having full blepharoplasty, however, are significant. Consider having both done at once.

the ear and face area to prevent contamination. For both upper and lower lids, the incision lines are carefully marked before anesthesia. Many surgeons prefer to do this with the patient sitting up. The upper- and lower-lid incisions may vary somewhat depending on the extent and location of flaccid skin. Both incisions generally extend into the crow's feet at the edge of the eye and are amazingly imperceptible after healing when done skillfully. Blepharoplasty is most frequently performed under local anesthesia, although some surgeons prefer general anesthesia. If a local anesthetic is used, the solution is injected with a small hypodermic needle beneath the eyelid skin.

The operation usually begins with the upper eyelid; skin approximately one-half inch wide and one and one-half inches long is removed. Then small pockets of fatty tissue are removed. This makes the eye much more alert looking (see the following before and after photos). The skin is stitched with sutures; most will be removed in three or four days. The lower-lid procedure replicates many of the same steps taken for the upper lid. The incision is directly below the lower lashes and heals to become invisible.

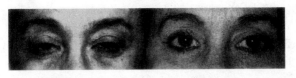

Presurgery eyes (left) show signs of aging. Final results (right) can be dramatic, giving a refreshed appearance to the face. (Source: Dr. Gregory LaTrenta)

Postoperative expectations:

To minimize postoperative swelling and discoloration, iced compresses are applied for 24 hours and must be continued slavishly for optimum results. The patient rests with the head elevated to further minimize swelling of the eyelids. Periodically, ointment is placed in the eyes and over the incision lines to protect the eye and minimize crusting of the suture line.

Bright Idea
Nearly everyone is able to resume normal activities quickly following an eye job (but no bending or lifting should be done). If you feel fine and want to get out, buy the largest pair of sunglasses you can find, pop on a hat, and go for it. Most people won't really notice.

There is usually little pain, but do expect some discomfort. Severe eye pain suggests the possibility of a complication. Most patients experience tightness, especially in the lower lids, for several weeks as the sutures heal and tighten. If the operation was performed in a hospital, the patient is usually discharged on the morning after the surgery with instructions to continue applying iced compresses. Ointment is applied to the suture lines three or four times a day and placed in the eye at night. If the eyes are dry, artificial tears are used as often as necessary and as directed by your doctor. At the time of discharge, the eyelids are frequently swollen and discolored. Much of this discoloration disappears in seven to ten days but may linger longer.

Remember, several stitches (at the outer lid) are left in place until the fifth day. This is often the point of maximal tension on the suture line, and early removal could possibly cause uneven healing. Don't be surprised if temporary blurring of vision lasts for several days. It can be minimized by keeping the eye moist with artificial tears. Occasionally other types of eye drops may be necessary, but only your surgeon must advise you on this.

Excessive skin removal during blepharoplasty can result in complications. In the upper lid, this may cause inability to close the eye (*lagophthalmos*). The amount of skin excision in the upper lid is planned so that after closure of the wound, the eyes do not close completely. By the morning after surgery, however, complete closure should be possible.

Excessive removal of lower lid skin may result in an *ectropion,* which is a pulling away of the lid from the eye. This problem is difficult to correct, so expect a top surgeon to be conservative when performing lower lid blepharoplasty. It is better to have several residual wrinkles in the lower lid than to have an ectropion result. Residual fine wrinkling of skin of the lower lid can often be improved by a chemical peel or laser resurfacing done several months after the blepharoplasty.

Common name: brow lift (coronal lift)
What it does: Smooths forehead frown lines and vertical frown lines between brows, and restores a more youthful arch to eyebrows
Price range: $4,500 to $7,000
Operation duration: Two to three hours
Anesthetic: Local with sedation or general
The procedure:
Sagging of the brow is a common accompaniment of facial aging. This drooping tends to be most marked in the outer half of the brow. It is a major factor in creating the hooded appearance of the upper lid that tends to obscure the edge of the eyelid. It usually produces a sad or tired look, and an eye job alone will not take care of the problem. In some cases, surgery on the upper lid actually pulls the brow down a bit on some patients. The normal brow lies 10 to 12 millimeters above the edge of the upper eyelid and the highest point of its arch is between the outer edge of the eyelids and the pupil.

Unofficially...
To test if your brow has drooped with aging, locate the bony ridge above your eyebrow (the top plane of your eye socket). See if the eyebrow remains on or above this ridge when you relax your appearance. Or you can elevate your brow by gently pulling upward with a finger to see if a more youthful arch improves your appearance.

The height and shape of the brow varies among individuals.

The function of the eyebrows is to assist the lids in protecting the eye. In response to irritants and other noxious substances, the lids close and the eyebrows contract, producing a squint. Brow lifts offer other advantages besides the obvious improvement in the position and shape of the brow. Most brow-lift procedures eliminate or improve the crow's feet at the outside corner of the eye.

There are several different brow-lift procedures. A general principle of brow surgery is that elevation increases when the incision is closer to the brow. Thus the operation utilizing an incision directly over the brow produces a greater brow lift than incisions in the hairline. Unfortunately, the resulting scar is more noticeable.

Although a sagging brow typically is not corrected by the standard face-lift operation, slight degrees of brow sagging may frequently be remedied during the operation by extending dissection into the temple.

There are two possible procedures; each varies by the length of the incision:

- A hairband incision—one that travels practically from ear to ear

- A less invasive endoscopic brow lift that usually makes two or more smaller incisions in the hairline above the brow

The endoscopic procedure usually takes one to two hours; the surgical team includes your doctor and anesthesiologist, a surgical nurse, and possibly another technician. Done this way, the brow lift is, for many patients, a less invasive, more effective procedure than the traditional open surgical method,

Watch Out!
Injury to the branch of the facial nerve that moves the forehead is possible during this brow surgery. Be absolutely certain that the surgeon you choose is experienced in doing brow surgery and familiar with nerve placement.

with its headband incision spanning from ear to ear. The endoscopic approach uses four or five small incisions in the scalp. Through these incisions, the forehead skin is elevated and the eyebrows are freed up from their attachment to the orbital bone. The doctor views the anatomy and procedure on a television screen. This procedure allows the eyebrows to be repositioned at a higher level on the forehead. The eyebrow elevation is maintained in position by using special sutures or miniscrews in the scalp incision. The screws or sutures are removed once the eyebrows have healed in their new position—usually two or more weeks after surgery. At the time of the eyebrow lift, the frown muscles between the eyebrows can be weakened or removed (as they can be with a traditional coronal lift).

The forehead lift is usually performed as an extension of the face-lift procedure but may be performed as a separate operation. When done with a face lift, incisions continue above the ear to meet in the center of the scalp one to two inches behind the hairline, or the surgeon employs endoscopic surgery. The forehead skin and attached frontalis muscle are elevated from the scalp to the level of the eyebrows. A portion of the frontalis muscle is usually removed at this time. The forehead skin is then stretched into its proper position, excess skin is removed, and the incision closed with sutures. In addition to improving forehead wrinkles, the forehead lift elevates eyebrows, re-creating an arching, youthful appearance, as seen in the following photos. This additional correction seems to be one of the most popular reasons for having the endoscopic forehead surgery.

Bright Idea
First introduced in the early 1990s, the endoscopic eyebrow or forehead lift was the first cosmetic procedure that used endoscopy. If you're thinking of the endoscopic approach, find a skilled surgeon who has performed brow endoscopy for several years.

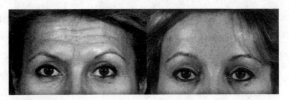

Vertical and transverse nasal frown lines can be corrected during the forehead lift by resection of the muscles that cause these wrinkles. (Source: Dr. Gregory LaTrenta)

Postoperative expectations:

In some cases, patients describe an odd sensation: The top of the head feels as if one were wearing an extremely tight ski cap. Other patients report significant swelling or some mild pain and discomfort. However, there should be little, if any, sharp or intensely throbbing pain. A sensation of pressure or tightness may be apparent for five to seven days. Mild pain-relieving medications are given as necessary. If they don't relieve the discomfort, alert your surgeon. In general, you should stay as quiet as possible, keep your head elevated, and avoid stooping over in the first month or so.

Possible complications:

The complications are rare and, if any, similar to those of a face lift—such as hematoma formation and unusual swelling. Injury to the facial nerves and loss of sensation may be long term. (Short-term numbness is likely to follow most brow-lift surgery.) The patient's healthy hair and hairline must be able to disguise the incision and eventual scar. Hair loss, though atypical, can result where the incisions are placed if the hair follicle has been damaged. Occasionally the brow may be overcorrected, resulting in an unattractive, surprised expression, and some asymmetrical results have been reported as well.

To reduce future frown lines on the brow, some surgeons remove a portion of the frown muscle or sever the nerve supply to the muscle during the operation. In extreme cases, the resulting lack of forehead animation often appears stoic and unnatural. Also, motion of the eyebrows, frequently an important element of happy facial expression and surprise, is usually impaired by this procedure. In many cases, the eyebrows gradually sag after this procedure, resulting in a second deformity that requires correction.

Common name: Botox (botulism toxin)

What it does: Paralyzes muscles that create wrinkles
Price range: $500 to $750 per injection
Operation duration: Minutes, after sedation
Anesthetic: Mild local sedation
The procedure:
The skin is wiped with a numbing agent; also a *sublingual tranquilizer* (placed under the tongue to dissolve) may be prescribed. After 20 minutes or so, the doctor, using a thin needle, injects botulism toxin. The liquid spreads to certain clusters surrounding the injection, typically in the forehead area, paralyzing the muscles that cause wrinkle damage. Some doctors have used Botox to eliminate deep brow furrows, crow's feet, and minimize the vertical cords of the neck. In some cases deep furrows are minimized immediately. Botox appears most useful for eliminating the vertical lines between the eyebrows, causing the person's expression to relax and appear less angry. The desired paralysis is generally temporary and lasts six months or so.

Postoperative expectations:
Virtually painless, the patient is immediately ambulatory but must remain inactive, with the head

upright, for several hours. This will help prevent the solution from drifting into undesirable areas. (If you're remotely concerned about moving your head unnecessarily, a neck brace can be prescribed to restrict movement.)

Possible complications:

Although most procedures have reportedly gone off without a hitch, some cases of drooping eyelids, asymmetrical corrections, and other sagging features have been reported. Apparently the first injection is the most effective. After that, the muscle may become inured to the toxin. Other doctors, in the absence of long-term studies, fear the muscle may become permanently damaged and lose its functionality. Controversy still surrounds the use of Botox, with some experts calling for the application to be reserved for treating serious facial tics.

Cost efficiencies

There are some benefits to undergoing several procedures at once. Time is better utilized, since recovering from a face lift and an eye job require about the same postoperative rest period. There are also cost savings: Anesthesia, operating room fees, and other medical expenses become less costly when several procedures are done at once. Here are some approximate average savings, based on national fees. Your expenses may be higher or lower, depending on who your surgeon is and where you live.

- Lower-face lift: $4,700
- Complete eye job: $2,900
- Brow lift: $2,800
- All three procedures: $8,500 as a package; $10,400 if done separately

- Upper lip resurfacing: $1,700
- Combined with lower-face lift: $5,500 as a package; $6,400 if done separately
- Lower-face lift and complete eye job: $6,500

Just the facts

- Face lifts remain one of the most effective methodologies for rejuvenating one's appearance.

- Finely etched lines near the eye or above the upper lip often respond well to skin resurfacing.

- Collagen or fat injection can smooth wrinkles.

- Eyes often show the first signs of aging, especially when "hooding" occurs in the upper lid; blepharoplasty is one of the more effective measures taken to rejuvenate a face.

- Scheduling several facial procedures at one time can save you money, but if you're unsure about accepting a totally new look, it may be better to undergo only one correction at a time.

GET THE SCOOP ON...
Understanding male-specific variables ▪ Getting
the best from a face lift ▪ Other anti-aging
approaches for men ▪ What men must know
about liposuction ▪ Penile enhancement

Special Surgical Considerations for Men

I t wasn't that long ago—perhaps a decade or two—when women made most doctor appointments for men and handled their other health issues, too. American men, it seemed, just didn't bother with those details. In fact, the purchase of nearly 85 percent of male grooming products and clothing was made for men by women. But now the dynamics have reversed. Growing readership in such magazines as *GQ, Details,* and *Men's Health* indicate how much more aware and involved men are becoming in their own well-being.

As men take responsibility for their own health-care choices, a growing number are also exploring cosmetic surgery. Certainly our national obsession with physical fitness proves that men of all ages can cultivate a lean body through a disciplined regime. Paul Newman, nearly 70 years old, defies any preconception of the average septuagenarian.

To a degree, the intense competition in the work force has fueled the popularity of cosmetic surgery

161

for men. I've seen how airline pilots, construction engineers, salesmen, and a variety of other workers have incorporated simple, one-day procedures into very busy schedules. Without much fanfare, they return to work looking more rested and feeling a renewed sense of confidence.

I've come to appreciate how terrific the benefits can be after interviewing, over the past two years, many men who have opted for cosmetic changes. Invariably, most men feel instantly recharged. They seem to seize each day with a new feeling of energy. Their previously flagging confidence, sometimes undermined by younger workers, is replaced by solid self-esteem.

If you wonder if cosmetic surgery is right for you, this chapter explains some of the ways men are seeking to improve their appearance. You'll get the details that will help you ask cogent and meaningful questions. Cosmetic surgery for men does vary from women. This chapter is devoted to those procedures that are male-exclusive or those that are adjusted for the male anatomy. To be sure, several cosmetic procedures such as eyelid surgery, nose surgery, and facial-implant surgery are performed essentially the same way for men and women (these are covered elsewhere in this book).

You always knew you were different . . .

You're rugged. You have more skin elasticity than women. Your tissue tends to be more sinewy. Cosmetic surgeons cite several male-specific variables that make performing cosmetic surgery on men different from performing it on women. While not 100 percent true for all men, in general, they:

- Require more anesthetic
- Experience greater blood loss

- Have less patience with the total process
- Are unable to adequately rest during recovery
- Insist on driving themselves home after surgery
- Disregard postoperative requirements
- Have a lower threshold for pain

Certain procedures are typically adapted for the male anatomy. While a man's age and health play a role in the quality of the outcome, how much hair he has, muscle definition, level of body fat, and other male-specific variables may affect how a technique can be used and what scarring is likely to develop. To ensure the best results, find a surgeon who has a strong male clientele supported by a solid, time-proven track record. You can also better evaluate your potential results by obtaining several before and after photos of male patients.

Getting the most from your face lift

If you are planning facial surgery (which may also somewhat improve the neck area), your doctor will evaluate your entire head-face-neck region. As a man, you have fewer styling options to minimize scars. Be certain you and your surgeon have discussed questions such as:

- Is your hairline receding?
- How full are your sideburns?
- Does your beard-growing skin extend up the cheeks or down the neck?
- Do you have any existing facial scars?
- Is your skin sun-damaged?
- Is your neck skin flaccid and loose?
- Exactly where will the incisions be placed?

If you are balding or have thinning hair, you'll need the best surgical artistry to hide any head

Unofficially...
A 1991 research study indicated that men have a higher level of dissatisfaction than women do following cosmetic surgery. Why? Men often expect perfection rather than prepare themselves for realistic results. Be certain the risks, recovery time, and other issues are carefully explained. Know where the incisions will be placed on your body.

incisions. This is especially crucial in the temple area where most of the incisions are done. The temple area is very visible to the eye and is likely to reflect light from many angles. On a well-executed face lift, after healing has transpired, a man should perceive no noticeable scarring. The thin incision in front of your ear should be virtually invisible, and the rugged muscles that control the chin and cheek area must appear relaxed, not artificially pulled.

Common name: face lift (facioplasty)

What it does: Eliminates mild sagging, modifies nose-to-mouth smile lines, generally improves the tone of the lower face

Price range: $3,500 to $15,000

Operation duration: Three to six hours

Anesthetic: Usually local, but many doctors prefer general anesthetic if they are doing supplemental surgeries

The procedure:

The incisions for face-lift surgery are commonly placed in the hairline as well as in front of the ear, under the chin, and in other areas where the scars can be expected to heal very well and where they are less conspicuous. For men, this is the most crucial aesthetic decision. If your ears protrude, the incisions behind the lobe may be very apparent for some time and the healing skin, which can be flaky and crusty for several weeks or more, will be visible. Discuss with your surgeon whether sutures or staples will be used and how the sutures will be made. Where will the incisions be made to anchor the newly pulled tissue? If you color your hair, be sure to do this several days before surgery since it will be at least four to six weeks before you can apply any coloring chemicals to your healing scalp.

After receiving the anesthetic, the facial area is cleaned with antiseptic solution and sterile cloths, and other surgical drapes are placed around the face to prevent contamination. The hair, too, is soaked with an antiseptic. With your before photos displayed for reference—these will include frontal and side shots—the surgeon will use a surgical marking pen to indicate all incision lines. Your face-lift incision is likely to begin in the natural crease in your sideburn area. Many men have a natural fold right where the earlobe and cheek meet. At the ear lobe, the incision continues around the ear's back, ascending in the crease between the ear and what's known as the *mastoid* area. (Tap behind your ear to feel the natural swelling, a small bony hill known as the mastoid.) At the top of the ear, the incision curves backward into the hairline. For some men, the incision extends into the temple hair, generally curving slightly forward much like a modified "s." The surgeon may adjust this basic incision depending on your general facial muscle tone, hairline, and natural skin folds.

Facioplasty incisions seek to camouflage scars on men while permitting surgeons flexibility to manipulate the underlying tissue. In some men, incisions go behind the earlobe extending up behind the ear to the center muscle, and then diagonally back into the scalp behind the ear.

After the incision is made in the temple area, a dissection follows just beneath the skin and skin fat, continuing to the fold between the lip and the cheek, and down to the midline of the neck. This is where the surgeon separates tissue and works expertly to minimize nerve damage. After the tissue is separated, it is lifted; this is called *undermining*.

Bleeding, a greater variable with men, is brought under control. By delving as far down as the chin and neck area, the surgeon is able to correct the sagging that comes with age.

The thin superficial muscle system is pulled backward in order to provide deeper support to facial tissue, particularly around the jaw. This muscle network is then sutured to the tissue just under the skin behind the ear. The skin is not reattached yet. Any fat on top of that area is removed to give a sleek, clean look. Then, six to eight sutures are placed down either side of the inside of the neck to secure the connective tissue and muscular layer before the skin is redraped. This creates the appearance of better face tone. Since men have a greater supply of blood to the face area, the surgeon must give considerable time to allow all of the blood vessels to coagulate. Any bleeding in the face may cause problems and potentially compromise results. The extra skin is carefully trimmed to eliminate pulling and wrinkling. The cheek skin is redraped and sutured to the ear. The skin behind the ear is pulled to help restore a firm jaw line.

As the skin is resutured, small tube drains may be placed in the neck area (behind or near the ear) in order to siphon any oozing. Expect blood and lymph to secrete through these drains as you rest upright in bed. A sterile dressing is applied and a helmet of bandages secures the head and neck area, pretty much hiding the black suture threads.

Postoperative expectations:

Your face will feel swollen and uncomfortable, but there should be no significant pain. Apply cold compresses vigilantly for the first 24 hours to minimize swelling and bruising. The day after surgery, any drains are removed along with the large bandage.

Watch Out!
If your newly pulled skin has hair, hair is likely to grow behind your ear. You may have to shave where you never had to prior to surgery.

You may feel a sensation of pressure. In general, you should keep as quiet as possible and avoid physical activity.

You'll be aware that you can't turn your head; this will mostly disappear within a few days. Most bruising goes through a predictable pattern of varying colors: red and blue bruises that may brown or turn jaundiced yellow before fading. The amount of bruising varies with each individual and that is why you must use cold compresses during the first 24 hours. Some patients go right into the final yellow stage while others show swelling and significant bruising. Unbelievably, many look almost normal within a few days.

A liquid or soft diet is usually prescribed for 48 hours to avoid use of chewing muscles. Your hair will be matted and feel sticky. Careful shampooing with a mild shampoo may be permitted as early as two days after the surgery, but follow your surgeon's protocol. The sutures in front of the ear are removed on the fifth postoperative day and you'll be able to see results better at that point. Sutures behind the earlobe and up into the hair line— temporal and mastoid sutures, which carry the pull of the newly toned face—are taken out near the seventh or tenth day. No sex is permitted for at least a week to keep your blood pressure normal. You are normally checked again a week later and then again four to six weeks after surgery. Be prepared for the possibility of odd swelling for the first week to 10 days. You may feel as if you have a small rock in the nape area or behind the ear. Some men report these swollen knobs can be itchy, uncomfortably warm, and annoying. Some swollen areas may have to be drained; others subside on their own.

Some important tips: You must keep your head upright! Do not bend over for three weeks or more. If you must bend, stoop at the knees, keeping your head upright.

Your surgeon will tell you when you can resume your normal athletic routine and what you can do. Many men return to work within two weeks. Remember: The healing process will continue internally for several more months. The face is usually numb in some areas because of inescapable injury to small nerve fibers that supply the skin. Regeneration of these fibers begins immediately and may be complete in six to twelve weeks, though numbness in varying degrees may continue for up to nine months to a year.

The best, fully realized results may not be apparent for several months or a year (see the following photos). After two weeks, however, you'll see improvement nearly every day until the face normalizes.

Unofficially...
Men underestimate recovery time and can inadvertently place pressure on the sutures. Vigorous activities should be avoided for one month—no jogging or gym workouts—because such exercise can temporarily elevate blood pressure and result in hemorrhage under the facial skin.

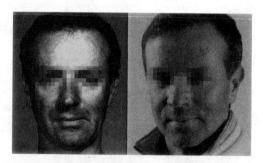

Lower facial sagging and aging can be minimized, as these typical before and after photos indicate. Minor neck improvement can be addressed as well, though significant neck aging requires its own remedial procedure. (Source: Dr. Gregory LaTrenta)

Another variation of the face lift, the endoscopic lift, often produces less bruising and fewer noticeable long-term scars. When the procedure is used before major aging has transpired, the operation is sometimes called a minilift. (Another procedure which is giving men good results—the new chin lipo/laser lift covered in Chapter 9—is known as the weekend lift.) However, results may be less dramatic.

Common name: face lift (endoscopic facioplasty)

What it does: Reduces lower facial sagging and signs of age

Price range: $7,000 and up

Operation duration: Three to four hours

Anesthetic: General

The procedure:

The endoscope is a telescope-like instrument that gives the plastic surgeon a window through which to see the anatomy. A fiber-optic light source and video camera are placed through a much smaller incision; the image is then transmitted from the endoscope to a television monitor. The surgeon is able to suture, staple, and rearrange tissue while watching his progress on the monitor. Because the resulting scars are much smaller than the scars from traditional facioplasty, men with thinning hair often benefit from endoscopy. The endoscopic face lift usually takes three to four hours; it is often more expensive due to the equipment and slightly larger surgical team: your doctor, the anesthesiologist, surgical nurses, and perhaps a nurse technician.

Endoscopic face-lift procedures are usually accomplished in two very different ways:

- The superficial approach
- The deeper lift approach

In the first approach, also called the subcutaneous technique, the skin, elevated through incisions at the hairline level, is pulled and pleated. At the hairline level above or behind the ear, the pleats slowly disappear over a period of several weeks. Because no tissue is undermined after the incisions, this really is a minilift. Men with deep facial creasing and other aging signs are not good candidates since the results are usually "mini" as well.

The second approach lifts the deep structure of the face by freeing up the overall original attachment and permitting the surgeon to re-anchor it to the facial bones. In many ways, some of the elements of the traditional face lift are deployed. However, gaining significant underlying tone is often more difficult. As with other face lifts, the tissue and muscle are then secured at a higher, pulled-back position. The end result of an endoscopic lift may be considerably less than that of the traditional face-lift procedure. If you wish a more dramatic, youthful result, you may wish to consider traditional facioplasty.

Postoperative expectations:

Most of the healing is less painful than a traditional face lift due to the smaller incisions and microscopic handling. Since the area is less traumatized, the patient may exhibit less bruising and swelling. However, most of the other postoperative expectations—swelling, keeping exercise to a minimum—prevail. And rigorous use of cold compresses is still necessary the first 24 hours.

Possible complications (both traditional and endoscopic):

Significant problems relating to traditional and endoscopic face lifts are infrequent. Because of the greater concentration of blood in the facial area, the most common complication is bleeding beneath the undermined facial skin. Most blood poolings are small and resolve spontaneously without consequence. Others are large enough to have the area aspirated with a large needle.

A serious complication can be the permanent loss of sensation along the cheek area (but remember, a numbing sensation may be experienced for up to a year). Patches of hair may be lost from the temporal area due to excessive tension on the facial skin or injury to hair follicles during the undermining process.

With men, surgically removing too much skin can cause tightly sutured wounds to be pulled by excessive tension on the undermined skin. Men should be aware that this potential result tends to yield an abnormally wide scar, which is more obvious on men.

Can't see your shirt collar?

Many men are concerned about the fatty or jowly area beneath the chin. In younger patients, generally men under 40 years of age, liposuction alone may correct the problem, though variations work well on older men, too. In some face-lift procedures, a light liposuction of a man's chin can make a significant difference. Some surgeons combine this step with a face lift. Other surgeons treat it as a separate procedure.

Common name: chin lift (liposuction)

What it does: Removes excess fat and skin to restore a more youthful-looking neck

Price range: $1,000 and up

Operation duration: Under one hour

Anesthetic: Typically local

The procedure:

A small incision is made under the chin, where frequently there's a natural crease already in place.

Bright Idea
Laser resurfacing or electrolysis can be used in some instances to do away with any new hair growth that may pop up in odd places following the redraping of skin. Discuss these options with your surgeon prior to surgery.

The surgeon slips in a siphoning device, called a cannula, and removes the fat by suction. (See Chapter 6 for details on the liposuction procedure.) A minor variation on this procedure—sometimes called *liposculpture*—uses a syringe. (Some doctors do call this the lunch-time lift when it's done as a single procedure. Don't plan on going back to work, though; schedule your surgery on Friday, rest over the weekend, and have the sutures removed on Monday.) If your chin skin is paper thin, a 2 mm to 3 mm syringe can extract fat. The syringe offers gentle aspiration and maximum control. Additionally, a small tool is necessary to remove fat in small amounts. It takes a little longer than liposuction, but uneven lumpiness that may occur with the larger cannula is less likely.

One postscript: Mildly loose neck skin can frequently be redraped in a face lift, creating a better profile. However, older patients (or men who've experienced major weight loss) may require a combination full face lift *and* full neck lift (the neck lift is covered in Chapter 9). Nevertheless, dramatic results can be seen in a simple one-day procedure, as shown in the following photos.

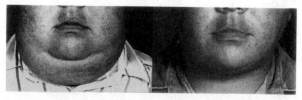

Because a man's collar and tie may accentuate a jowly area, a simple syringe procedure or, as in this case, more extensive liposuction can quickly give greater jaw definition and improve an out-of-shape appearance. (Source: Dr. Gregory LaTrenta)

Other anti-aging tricks for the male face

Refinishing treatments for facial skin can help diminish sun damage and give a man's complexion a smoother, more youthful appearance. If you can handle the healing time, usually two weeks or more, you can schedule time away from work or rearrange your schedule around a series of skin resurfacing techniques.

In most cases, men tend to wrinkle less than women because they have more *collagen* beneath the skin. Collagen is the major protein of connective tissue and contributes to the plumping beneath skin. The chemical peel—a form of chemosurgery—is a valuable technique for rejuvenating a man's face that has significant sun damage. The chemical peel, on the other hand, does not improve the general sagging of the skin of the face and neck. All peel candidates must be chosen exceptionally carefully.

Many men are unaware that medium to light chemical peels can offer good benefits. Perhaps a number of beauty ads and spa claims have imparted a too-feminine benefit to peels so men tend to exclude them as a realistic option. Here are two peels that work well on men:

- TCA (trichloracetic acid) burns off the entire epidermis and only the most superficial portion of the dermis.

- Glycolic acid, the mildest of peeling agents, removes only the outer layers of the epidermis.

Another peel made with phenol is often less suitable for men who lack the patience required by the significant postoperative follow-up and attention to recovery. All peels, including TCA and glycolic peels, produce a burn of the skin. Most peels, except full-face *deep* peels, are typically done on an outpatient basis. Peeling almost always causes a permanent decrease in skin pigmentation which is more noticeable in darker skins; the line between treated and untreated skin is often clearly evident, though TCA peels have reduced this considerably. A man's beard and shaving may eventually minimize any line.

Common name: face peel (chemosurgery)

What it does: Chemically burns the skin, minimizing superficial wrinkles, brown age spots, and other minor external signs of sun damage and aging

Price range: $300 to $5,000, depending on depth and type of peel

Operation duration: One hour (or less) to several hours

Anesthetic: Local or general, depending on depth and type of peel

The procedure:

Before a peel, the patient may be required to use certain topical medications to begin the exfoliation process. Right before the peel is applied, the face is carefully washed with surgical antiseptic. The skin is gently stretched during peel application so that the solution will uniformly coat the skin and the bottom of each fine wrinkle. Application continues into the hairline and eyebrows and up to the lips. Neck skin is not peeled because a high incidence of scarring and abnormal pigmentation are common. A very light solution, if any, is applied to eyelids since the skin is exceedingly thin and delicate. A burning sensation follows several seconds after each application. The patient, ambulatory afterwards, returns home and stays indoors to allow the crusting stage to begin.

Unofficially...
Apart from complexion color, the texture of the skin is also an important factor in selection of peel patients. Fair-skinned men with moist skin do better. Men with thick, oily skin are more apt to develop uneven skin pigmentation and are best served by very mild peels.

Postoperative expectations:

Approximately one-half hour after the peel is completed, the patient begins to experience a mild warm sensation, much like a very mild itching or burn. In very light peels, some men report little, if any, new sensation. Over the next few days, pin-sized whiteheads called *milia* frequently occur. These areas are caused by temporary obstruction of small glands of the facial skin and, in most cases, can be satisfactorily treated by gentle washing. Some milia must be opened with a sharp needle. You will not be able to shave until your surgeon advises you. It might be a week or less. Many men enjoy this scruffy respite; in some cases the new beard growth disguises the skin's transformation.

With all peels, except very mild glycolic solutions, a significant scaly crust forms and falls off, though afterward no treatment is necessary other than frequent gentle washing and application of a bland ointment to help retain skin moisture. With deep and medium peels, ointments containing cortisone-like agents are sometimes prescribed. However, after a chemical peel, be prepared for persistent redness much like a sunburn.

With very light peels, often procedures are done as a series, perhaps three or four sessions, extended over several weeks or months. Exposure to the sun must be carefully avoided for three to six months, and avoiding the sun altogether may prevent continual, excessive wrinkling.

Possible complications:

Problems can range from minor to severe and usually relate to uneven skin pigmentation results. In some cases, this is due to the unpredictability of certain skin types and may be beyond the direct control of the surgeon. Occasionally, areas of splotchy

Watch Out!
Permanent skin tags, blotches, and blemishes before the peel may be darker after the procedure. The best preventive measure is to remove them (through excision or laser) before a chemical peel.

hyperpigmentation develop after a chemical peel. Again, this problem occurs most frequently in men with dark complexions, but may also occur in light-skinned patients after sun exposure. Repeeling of the face often is necessary to correct this, but it may have to be delayed long after the first peel.

Some men may also wish to consider collagen injections, ultrapulsed laser treatments, or dermabrasion to rejuvenate skin. These are covered in Chapter 7, along with another facial rejuvenating procedure, the brow lift. While these procedures are much the same for men and women, with brow lifts a man's hairline and choice of surgeon are especially crucial for obtaining a good final result.

The benefits of liposuction for men

In the past few years, no plastic surgery technique has received more press—or more male customers—than liposuction. In the early '90s, barely 6,000 men had liposuction. By the end of the decade, it's likely the number will grow tenfold. Liposuction could become the number-one cosmetic procedure for men. (See Chapter 6 for a complete discussion on liposuction and how it works. I'll limit our discussion here to male-specific issues.)

Not just reducing—reshaping

Liposuction is revolutionary for men because it means anti-aging cosmetic surgery is no longer limited to facial procedures. Since men retain their skin elasticity longer than women do, and the areas of fat beneath the skin tend to be firmer with a somewhat greater concentration of vessels, liposuction can be exceptionally effective.

There are four variables that help shape the ideal male body:

- The anatomy is trim and athletic-looking.
- The shoulders and chest are broad.
- The abdomen is flat.
- The hip-thigh area tends to be narrow.

However, as men age, areas of fat tend to accumulate around the abdomen, the flanks ("love handles"), the breast area (a condition called *gynecomastia*), and along the chin and neck. Men sometimes seek liposuction to reduce these fatty areas that can be resistant to diet and exercise (see the following photos).

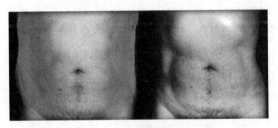

"Love handles" and a growing spread to the waistline respond well to major liposuction and show dramatic improvement. (Source: Dr. Gregory LaTrenta)

Traditional liposuction vacuums indiscriminately and the results can be less asymmetrical, less smooth. A new methodology, called UAL or ultrasound assisted liposuction (see Chapter 6) seems to work especially well on the male body in the fibrous areas that are male-specific, such as the back and the upper chest. This is because it uses a smaller cannula that can target the fat cells which have been liquefied by the ultrasonic wave.

Recovery issues for men
Although men seldom report pain when they talk about their plastic surgery, they will admit to some

discomfort after having liposuction. Some patients said it was much like being pummeled with a blunt instrument or having a bruised or broken rib.

Bright Idea
Ask your doctor if you can wear a pair of snug-fitting bike pants or bike shorts in place of the girdle.

All liposuction (even under the chin!) requires a tight bandage or other restrictive material that keeps the loose skin from moving. If you've had your abdomen done, be prepared for wearing adhesive foam under a skintight girdle. You'll keep this on the treated area(s) for about a week. Then you'll wear a tight girdle for four to six weeks more. Unfortunately, after a grueling day at work, you can't step out of this girdle—it must be worn around the clock! All men I interviewed reported that the elastic bandage, worn day and night, proved to be a constant annoyance.

The days and weeks immediately following your liposuction surgery are critical to obtaining a good final result. Follow your doctor's advice to the letter. It's very likely that his or her orders will include:

- Taking adequate time off from work
- Wearing bandages or tight compression garments religiously
- Getting enough bed rest
- Staying out of the sun
- Saying no to alcohol and cigarettes
- Avoiding strenuous activity, exercise, and sports for the first few weeks following surgery
- Abstaining from sex until you get the green light

Many plastic surgeons understand that it's practically impossible for men, who are programmed by society to be stoic, to remain in bed for very long. Few men, if any, accept help from others during recovery. We know men often deny their pain and feel foolish asking for help after surgery. Further, be prepared for depression in some form or another. It can be a deep funk or a fleeting bad day. To minimize mood swings, don't cut yourself off from loved ones or those who can offer help and comfort. Even the distraction of renting a good video with a friend can get you over the slump. Or it may prevent the slump entirely!

Some male patients I interviewed were not prepared for others noting the change. Do you tell or not tell? Are you going to clue coworkers in? The choice is yours. Many men are more comfortable discussing body issues than women, although this is changing as women become increasingly more comfortable with their bodies. Chapter 4 provides tips on how you may wish to deal with telling others.

One Arizona marketing executive, who in the course of three years had a tummy tuck, a neck lift, and UAL on his abdomen and thighs, says, "People knew I had lost weight. But they could not figure out exactly why I looked better." So he told them about his plastic surgery; most did not believe him. "But as soon as I told them, it became a nonissue that went away."

Breast reduction and potbelly liposuction

Some men have excess fat that accumulates in the breast area. For many men, this is a natural aspect of general aging, much like the potbelly that seems to show up in tandem with middle age. Apart from general aging, the condition can also be exacerbated by abuse of alcohol or by anabolic steroids or hormone treatment for prostate cancer.

In addition to older patients, very young men often elect breast reduction. When hormones surge in teenage years, almost half of young men have

Timesaver
Recovery from liposuction often startles men. Have a support person available— both physically and emotionally— for about a week after surgery. Men who reject help may have an especially difficult recovery, and are more predisposed to postoperative depression during the weeks following surgery. You'll see results a lot sooner.

some form of gynecomastia, an enlargement of the breast area. Fortunately, nearly 90 percent of these cases resolve in a year or two as the body adjusts to manhood. Surgery results can be significant.

Common name: fatty chest reduction (gynecomastia)

What it does: Removes extra fat or glandular tissue that imparts a female appearance to a male chest

Price range: $3,500 to $6,000

Operation duration: About two hours

Anesthetic: General

The procedure:

An incision is made in the lower half of the *areola*, the pink colored area surrounding the nipple, and, if the cause is excess fat, the fat is removed via liposuction. However, many men also have glandular tissue that must be excised in conjunction with liposuction. Scars heal well and in many cases are invisible. However, if the surgeon requires larger incisions to remove excess skin, these are likely to extend two to three inches down the side of each breast, but eventually should fade to pale. Drains may also be inserted, and a compression garment or elastic bandages are applied.

Postoperative expectations:

Since you'll have to wear a compression garment that restricts movement, scheduling the operation during hot weather can add to the inconvenience. If this procedure is performed by itself, typically on an outpatient basis, you will have a soreness that can be likened to extreme muscular pain that accompanies a super-rigorous workout. The difference, however, is that the pain may increase as you heal; it can easily last for a week or more. You may require a prescribed pain medication the first week and an

Bright Idea
Certain drugs, such as anabolic steroids or marijuana, in addition to being dangerous and/ or illegal, can contribute to a flabby, flaccid male chest. Eliminating such drugs can often cause the swelling to subside. A simple exercise program can then impart greater definition.

over-the-counter analgesic for another week or until the pain diminishes. Most normal activity and day-to-day movement—*not* exercise—can be resumed within a few days, though you may not feel up to traveling. You'll be able to drive a car after three days or so. Your doctor will advise when you may return to the gym or undertake manual labor. Walking is one of the best ways to get your system going, but stay off the bicycle.

Possible complications:

A crater-like irregularity that pushes the breast inward, sometimes called a *saucer deformity,* can develop. Choose a surgeon experienced in the treatment of gynecomastia who will know how to feather the dissection area, thereby reducing the inward pull that may result. Smokers in particular may develop noticeable scars and experience skin loss, including the nipple. Asymmetry occurs often, but this usually resolves over time. If not, ask your surgeon *before* the operation if a corrective follow-up procedure is possible. Sun worshippers run the risk of darkening the scar; you must block incisions from harmful UV rays.

Common name: mini-tummy tuck (mini-abdominoplasty)

What it does: Diminishes or removes potbelly bulge
Price range: $2,000 to $4,000 or more
Operation duration: About two and a half hours
Anesthetic: Usually local with sedation
The procedure:

The "pot" area is marked with a surgical marker in concentric circles much like a target. Once the largest amount of fat from the bull's eye is removed, the surgeon works slowly toward the edges of the target. Like any highly skilled performer, a good surgeon makes the procedure appear simple, but liposuction isn't. A full abdominoplasty or major tummy tuck may be chosen by men who have hanging abdominal skin (usually the result of massive weight loss), large amounts of fat, loose abdominal muscles, and/or neglected hernias. It is a major surgical procedure that removes excess fat, tightens the muscles of the abdominal wall, and trims the waistline. With UAL, a skilled surgeon may be able to sculpt the body. Men who have a full abdominoplasty are often surprised by the recuperation time. Some patients aren't able to return to work for up to four weeks after surgery.

Postoperative expectations:

Even though the operation is called a "mini," you will likely be limited in what you can do during the first week. Guided by your physician, you can expect a progressive return to normal activity in about two to six weeks. A few patients remark that the pain is greater than anticipated, although most find the pain is as anticipated. There can be swelling and bruising, but this tends to subside reasonably quickly. Some male patients note that it may take some time for the new shape to settle in, although results are obvious almost immediately.

Possible complications:

As with all surgeries, there can be problems with healing, infection, and hemorrhaging. If too much fat is removed, the skin may not heal properly. But in most minor fat removal procedures, there are few serious complications.

Washboard chest and other body sculpting

In recent years, plastic surgeons have developed ways of improving muscle contour with cosmetic

Moneysaver
Men with good skin elasticity who have only a moderate amount of excess abdominal fat may benefit from a diligent sit-up program. A simple abdominal training apparatus can deliver initial results within weeks if the exercise routine is followed rigorously—and it can cost under $100, versus thousands of dollars for liposuction.

implants and sculpting techniques. A small number of doctors have begun offering their male patients abdominal etching, a new liposuction technique that creates a muscular, rippled appearance in the abdominal area.

Men who consider cosmetic muscle enhancement should keep in mind that these procedures are still relatively new. You absolutely must seek out a board-certified plastic surgeon who has received adequate training and experience in these methods. Similarly, pectoral implants can also be used to provide heft to the existing pectoral muscles of healthy men. However, this body sculpting can be executed only by a surgeon with great aesthetic sense and enormous liposuction skill. Keep reading for some tips that will help ensure that you are not ripped off, compromised, or hurt by unskilled hands.

UAL experience is critical

Do not submit yourself to UAL surgery performed by someone who's just learning the technique. Make sure the doctor you choose has adequate training and experience in doing the procedure; never opt for a doctor who does fewer than a dozen procedures a year. If you need to travel to a major metro area or leading hospital, do so. To find the best UAL-proficient surgeon, seek a doctor who's been performing liposuction for several years and UAL for more than one year. If you are thinking about one of the newer sculpting approaches, you must seek a qualified surgeon who does the same lipo procedure you want at least four or more times a week. Performing a procedure that many times indicates an ongoing expertise and shows that the surgeon is known—and sought after—for that type of surgery.

Speak with several male patients who have
undergone the same procedure you're considering.
Of course, you'll be referred to satisfied customers.
Still, do ask them the same questions about pain,
recovery time, complications, technical details, and
cost to see if their answers match what the doctor
told you. Here are some other factors that can contribute to a more successful procedure:

- A hospital, not an in-office surgery facility, is the
  ideal setting for large-volume liposuction in case
  complications arise.

- If a doctor operates from an office, ask if the
  facilities are state of the art.

- Also, if the doctor uses an anesthesiologist, be
  sure to check his or her credentials as well (see
  Chapter 3).

- Ask if the operating room or the surgical site
  carries a "Four-A rating." This means that the
  facility meets the inspection requirements of
  the American Association for Accreditation of
  Ambulatory Surgery Facilities (verify by contact-
  ing them at 1202 Allanson Road, Mundelein,
  Illinois 60060; 1-847-949-6058). Finally, make
  sure the facility that serves you complies with
  federal, state, and local codes as well as association standards (for example, all doctors using
  the facility must have hospital privileges at least
  at one local hospital).

Making the penis appear larger

In 1995, in a study of 60 healthy males, researchers
at the University of California-San Francisco found
that, on average, the penis when erect measured 5.1
inches in length and 4.9 inches in circumference.
These researchers believe that many American men

are being duped about penile augmentation. They presented their findings at a medical convention in Las Vegas. The controversy surrounding this procedure continues today. What did the research show? First, the study sought to answer, exactly what is too small? Also, did these men really need an implant? Below normal is estimated to be an erect penis under 2.8 inches in length or less than 3.5 inches in girth, according to these University of California researchers. Their study indicates that none of the 60 men studied had penises smaller than that and, at the very most, only one in 50 men had a penis that is actually smaller than the normal range. Many plastic surgeons agree that very few men are candidates for penile augmentation; the operation should be reserved for men who have suffered traumatic injuries.

Are surgeons taking advantage of male insecurities by charging large fees and doing unnecessary penile surgical procedures? One researcher who participated in the University of California study, Hunter Wessells, a clinical instructor of urology at San Francisco General Hospital, believes the answer is yes. In fact, the research was initiated after several men sought help after having penile surgery and were unhappy with the results.

Dr. Gary Alter, a Beverly Hills urologist, vigorously defends the procedure. Dr. Alter has performed a few dozen of these procedures and suggests the unhappy outcomes are traceable to one or two bad doctors. (Reader beware!) Dr. Alter argues that any man with a self-esteem problem should go ahead and explore having the surgery, as long as the surgeon is qualified and gives him an honest assessment of what to expect. "It's done for self-esteem

Watch Out!
If penile enlargement is performed for purely cosmetic reasons, the procedure is not covered by insurance.

Watch Out!
It wasn't that long ago that doctors freely injected loose silicone into women's breasts. The results were both hideous and disastrous over the long term. Similarly, there's an absence of quantitative data relating to the safety of penile augmentation.

issues," Dr. Alter explains, just like a hair transplant, breast implant, or other plastic surgery. However, expectations, as with all cosmetic procedures, must be realistically assessed along with the risks. And like all relatively new procedures, the absence of long-term data may inadvertently minimize future complications.

Common name: penile enhancement

What it does: Makes the penis *appear* larger
Price range: $500 to $5,000
Operation duration: About one hour
Anesthetic: Generally local
The procedure:

There are two basic penile augmentation procedures that are gaining coverage in the media: fat injection and penile lengthening.

Like breast implants on normal-size women, the majority of these augmentation procedures are done on men with penises of normal size. The first procedure, fat injection, harvests the patient's own fat, which is injected into the penis to enhance its size. In some patients, injected fat lasts for several months or longer. In others, fat seemingly vanishes right away.

The second penile procedure is sometimes called the penis-lengthening operation. The penis itself is really not lengthened; the surgery creates an optical illusion. The net illusory gain can range from an inch to an inch-and-one-half. The procedure involves cutting the suspensory ligament of the penis at its attachment, close to the pubis. This gives the appearance that the penis is longer.

Postoperative expectations:

There is not enough individual male response to provide meaningful general guidelines for postoperative expectations. However, doctors urge each patient to seriously consider the possible risks. There has been little reported discomfort from those males who chose fat injections. Those who have undergone the penis lengthening procedure, however, have remarked on a mild tenderness for several days after surgery. This seems to fade quickly. Patients should refrain from having sex as your surgeon directs.

Possible complications:

The risks for both procedures are significant and similar. For fat injection, possible complications may include infection, skin loss, sensory loss, or loss of function. For the lengthening procedure, many of the same symptoms have been reported. But most important, the erect penis may be compromised by loss of the ligament support.

Due to the controversial nature of this cosmetic procedure, a number of top surgeons seriously question the need and long-term safety of this particular approach. As a reporter, I've come across a number of cautionary tales that give credence to their skepticism. Curious readers may wish to explore an article written by reporter John Taylor in *Esquire.* The article, *"The long, hard days of Dr. Dick,"* appeared in the September 1995, volume 124 issue and underscores the need for taking responsibility for any cosmetic medical treatment one elects to have.

Once again, it's critical to seek an evaluation from a qualified, board-certified plastic surgeon who is skilled in the area you are seeking to modify. And with penile enhancement, only a seasoned or expert plastic surgeon can help you assess the attending risks and evaluate your individual needs.

> "
> Penile augmentation is unproved to be safe and is unregulated. There are no long-term studies and the ASPRS strongly cautions against using fat to augment the penis. In general, results of fat injected to enhance *any* tissue varies considerably from person to person.
> —Research expert Hunter Wessells, a clinical instructor of urology at San Francisco General Hospital
> "

Just the facts

- Because of their facial features and general anatomy, men have different considerations for cosmetic surgery than women.

- Men can be good candidates for face lifts, but should consult with their surgeon to determine whether the hairline can be used to camouflage incisions.

- Anti-aging treatments such as chemical peels can help diminish sun damage and give a man's complexion a smoother, more youthful appearance.

- Liposuction is becoming a popular option for men who want to reshape their bodies.

- If you're interested in UAL liposuction, make sure the surgeon you choose has plenty of experience in this technique.

- Much of the new penile cosmetic surgery remains untested for long-term risks and results, but procedures can be effective for the right candidate and in the hands of an experienced, board-certified plastic surgeon.

GET THE SCOOP ON...
The challenges of performing cosmetic surgery
on the neck ▪ Determining which approach
is right for you ▪ Traditional procedures to
produce a smooth, youthful neck ▪ Removing
the turkey gobbler ▪ The weekend lift: a
controversial alternative to a face lift

Other Innovative Procedures

Chapter 9

The neck is a curious part of the human anatomy. Centuries ago, many European cultures viewed certain physical attributes as a measure of a one's station in life. For example, long, slimly tapered fingers belonged to aristocrats, skilled court musicians, or accomplished surgeons. A long, slender neck was another desirable, upper-class trait, as any Titian portrait suggests. A long neck permitted titled noblemen and kings to survey the battlefield and remain "heads and shoulders" above their minions.

Today, there is still no way to lengthen the neck, but the area can be made to appear more sleek and youthful through various cosmetic procedures. Most of these advances are fairly recent developments. Historically, improving the neck involved an aesthetic price: a visible scar. Some procedures obviate the scar, but not in all cases.

This chapter will tell you all you need to know about cosmetic procedures on the neck.

Traditional neck procedures

There are several cosmetic operations that address a flabby or wrinkled, even significantly aged neck. But each person's neck offers the surgeon a variety of challenges. These are best addressed by different surgical procedures. Which operation is right for you?

There is a wide range of highly individual neck sizes, shapes, and overall appearances. For example, many young people in their twenties have thin lines that practically circle the entire neck; these are typically hereditary and not due to aging. Other prospects in their thirties may have early signs of a turkey gobbler, a flabby pouch of fat that diminishes the line of the jawbone. And many people in their seventies—without cosmetic surgery—sport a trim neck that shows very little aging. So, indeed, age can be a factor, but other factors such as heredity and sun damage can play a role in the shape of your neck as well.

You can do your own evaluation by checking your full face and neck appearance in a mirror. Examine each side of your profile, too. Try to identify the conditions that a surgeon will evaluate. Most surgeons will assess four variables before determining the best approach:

- Overall skin tone in the neck region: Does it cling to the neck or hang loosely? Can you easily pull an inch with your fingertips? Does the excess skin bounce back or hang?

- Is there excessive fat accumulation under the chin or throughout the neck? Has your jaw definition been lost or does your lower neck protrude or hang over a shirt or blouse collar?

- When you relax your expression, are the neck muscles (called the platysma muscles) toned or do they appear to droop, forming two bridle-like, stringy cords on each side?

■ A surgeon will also address the location of your hyoid bone, the U-shaped bone in the neck that supports the tongue. In many profiles, the end of the chin thrust lines up (more or less) with the tip of the nose. If the placement recedes backward, the neck tends to be shorter. As fat gathers there—even in slim people—the jaw line loses definition. In very young patients, recessed hyoid bones can create the appearance of a premature double chin. In these cases, a chin implant (see Chapter 11) may be the best remedy for the neck's appearance. As with face lift and other forms of cosmetic surgery, the supplemental operations designed to correct the aging neck may be performed either in an outpatient surgical facility or in a hospital operating room. Although most such operations are performed under local anesthetic, some surgeons use a general anesthetic.

Treatments for the neck range from mild chemical peels to the more complicated removal of the turkey gobbler. If it appears that your skin surface is the culprit, consider a mild chemical or laser treatment (see Chapter 7). However, if the appearance of your neck appears to be compromised by slack muscles or very loose skin, even a simple double chin, then the following procedures are more likely to address your concerns.

Redraping the neck as an adjunct procedure

Some neck aging, typically mild signs, can be addressed in a face-lift procedure. This correction is often known as a neck redrape. During the face lift, the neck tissue is widely undermined through the

Timesaver
After 40 years of age or so, sagging of the neck skin is almost always accompanied by laxity of the facial skin. In many cases, a modified, simple neck lift can be performed in conjunction with the face lift. These tucks work best to correct mild cases of neck aging and can save recovery time and money.

incisions in front of the ears. This allows the entire area to be lifted maximally. The shape and location of the tension bearing incisions behind each ear (and in the hairline) are then typically sutured carefully to conceal or camouflage scarring. These incisions pick up the slack of sagging neck skin. Most surgeons believe that suturing the superficial neck muscles with stitches helps produce a more effective neck lift.

During this redrape procedure, some surgeons also remove small amounts of supplemental fat through a small incision under the chin, either excising it with scissors or through liposuction. In some cases, the edges of the platysma muscle responsible for the bridled appearance can be approached through this incision and sutured together, or the muscles themselves can be trimmed and then sutured together. The price for this supplemental surgery can be inclusive in the face lift, or it can cost up to $7,000 or so. Each surgeon and each individual case dictate cost variables.

Neck resculpting

Perhaps your neck has begun to trouble you enough to consider some surgical treatment, but you don't want a face lift. If you don't opt for a face lift, a simple neck procedure, detailed below, can create a noticeable improvement. This approach is best for making moderate or conservative corrections. Also, as I mentioned earlier in this chapter, the position of the hyoid bone may limit the surgeon's ability to improve the neck's appearance. Since the surgeon cannot change the hyoid position in a neck tuck, you may wish to consider a chin implant as well.

Common name: Light neck sculpting

What it does: Removes fat; in some cases, excess loose neck skin can be tucked

Price range: $3,500 to $5,000

Operation duration: Under two hours

Anesthetic: Local, or local with sedation (MAC) if significant redraping is required

The procedure:

While this procedure often works best on patients who are 45 years of age and under, I've seen a number of remarkable results enjoyed by older candidates.

After sedating the patient and surgically cleaning the area, the surgeon places a small incision under the chin. In most cases this cut will heal to become imperceptible. Usually only one or two sutures are necessary to close the incision.

Once the neck is opened and bleeding is brought under control, pockets of excess neck fat are removed. These can be suctioned out using a hand-held aspirator. Some surgeons prefer a small liposuction cannula to treat double chins. In young patients, the skin typically rebounds so there's no need to nip or tuck (see the following photos). (A compressive surgical dressing is necessary, however, to encourage tightening during the recovery.) In other cases, a certain amount of sagging skin can be excised and then tucked up. Different combinations of procedures are used, depending on the problem, age of patient, and desired aesthetic outcome.

As with a number of neck procedures, after the fat is suctioned away, some surgeons also seek to tighten slightly sagging platysma muscles. If the surgeon begins with a tumescent injection, as described in Chapter 6, bleeding is minimized, and, once the skin swells, isolated fat can be more readily removed. This reduces postoperative bruising and swelling in many cases.

Watch Out!
Do not use age to predict your aesthetic success. For many neck alterations, the best outcome can be traced to a healthy degree of skin elasticity and your inherited position of the hyoid bone.

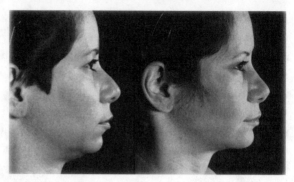

A slimmer, more youthful-looking neck is evident following corrective surgery. This patient also elected to have nose reshaping.
(Source: Dr. Gregory LaTrenta)

It's worth repeating (since many patients apparently dismiss this possibility in their preoperative
consultation): If skin has lost elasticity and will not
rebound successfully on its own, this loose skin
may have to be cut. The resulting scar may be much
more apparent. Discuss the possibility of scar formation with your surgeon during your consultation.

Postoperative expectations:

The degree of discomfort varies with each patient.
In general, most patients experience an uncomfortable tightness or tenderness of the neck immediately upon awakening—this discomfort dissipates
over the first few hours or days. Turning the neck
may be difficult; other patients feel virtually no discomfort. Cold compresses and a mild painkiller prescribed by the physician should effectively manage
the first 48 hours. After that, most patients can
resume mild activity. Within a week, sometimes less,
many return to a nearly full schedule.

Possible complications:

Significant problems are infrequent, but the most
common occur when there is bleeding beneath the

skin. (Remember, there's a greater concentration of blood vessels in the facial area.) Most blood pooling is small and resolves spontaneously without consequence. Other collections may have to be aspirated with a large needle. Infection is rare and can be treated with antibiotics. As a patient, be aware of any significant redness or unusual sharp pain that does not go away. A number of patients are surprised at a lingering numbness or the inability to comfortably raise the chin to look upward. This varies from patient to patient and is likely to totally disappear within a month or two.

The turkey gobbler

In cases of extreme fat accumulation, severe sun damage, or other factors such as aging and heredity, a distinct formation called a turkey gobbler may appear on the neck—a loose, hanging pocket that often moves when a person talks. This extreme condition often requires a different correction, and the procedure is a more extensive operation. Sometimes this irregularity is best treated in conjunction with a face lift but not done at the same time. A number of surgeons postpone gobbler removal six to eight weeks after the face lift. The skin tension in the neck that results from the face lift might widen the scars if both procedures are performed simultaneously. There's another reason (and patient benefit) to postponing a neck procedure until several weeks after a face lift: The extent to which neck appearance has been remedied can be more accurately assessed. Any other correction can be planned and discussed at that time. If your surgeon suggests this approach, be sure to understand the rationale behind this recommendation.

Bright Idea
Postponing neck surgery until after your face lift also has an upside. In some cases, the neck responds better than anticipated and patients feel no need for additional surgery.

Common name: Turkey gobbler removal

What it does: Gives a more youthful appearance by removing the wobbling pocket of fat and tightening slack skin beneath the chin

Price range: $5,000 to $9,000

Operation duration: Varies, but typically under two hours

Anesthetic: Usually local with sedation (MAC), unless done with other procedures

The procedure:

Incisions of various configurations have been designed by top surgeons, and your type of incision must be individually evaluated. It may be directly under the chin or in a natural fold. In some cases, the gobbler itself has pulled to such an extent that a natural crease or several lines have formed directly beneath the chin. Some surgeons use one or several natural creases to accommodate the incisions. Others employ a single incision that may extend along a major portion of the jaw line beneath the chin. The incisions must permit the surgeon adequate access to flaccid platsyma muscles to perform the major correction.

Some surgeons restitch the gobbler muscles back to their original position. Others feel that partial removal of the muscles yields better results.

Through the incisions, fat deposits below the chin and throughout the neck can be accessed to create a slimmer contour. Because the overlying skin has been stretched beyond the configuration of the new contour, a smaller redrape must be created. The surgeon will excise this loose, thin, and crepey skin to achieve an optimum result, as shown in the following before and after photos. This is why your final scar may not be so easily camouflaged. The scar must be long enough so that the redraped skin will heal in a flat, smooth fashion. If the incision is too short, the new skin will pleat and pucker as it is pulled up and restitched in place. Your final scar is dependent on your own wound healing capability and other individual factors.

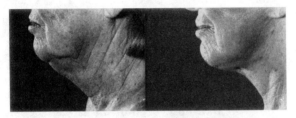

Extreme neck sagging and the accompanying turkey gobbler attribute can be dramatically altered, as these typical before and after photographs indicate. (Source: Dr. Gregory LaTrenta)

Postoperative expectations:

A tight chin strap or binding bandage remains in place for at least the first 24 hours. Often this chin strap or a modified version is worn until swelling subsides or as your surgeon directs. There's no doubt about it: For the first couple of days, nearly all patients experience an uncomfortable, dull pain and discomfort. Swallowing may be difficult for some early on in recovery. For this reason, a soft or liquid diet is prescribed to eliminate chewing. Bruising and swelling vary according to the correction and each patient's own response. A sensation of pressure or an uncomfortable tightness is common below the chin, but this tends to diminish in days and adjustment is rapid for most people. If prescribed painkillers don't relieve the discomfort, alert your surgeon. In general, you should stay as quiet as possible until your doctor advises increased activity.

Bright Idea
Keep a tiny, clip-on lamp attached to your book so you can read and doze without having to twist your torso to turn off your bedside lamp.

You may not be able to swivel your head, but this will mostly disappear within a few days. Most bruising goes through a predictable pattern of varying colors: red and blue bruises that may turn brown or jaundiced yellow before fading. Remarkably, some patients look almost normal within a few days.

You are normally checked again a week later after the first suture removal and then for a final time four to six weeks after surgery.

Gradual resumption of simple activities is recommended; walking will help galvanize the healing process. However, don't bend over for three weeks or more. If you must, bend at the knees, keeping your head upright. Never lift anything heavy or strenuously place pressure on the sutures. Vigorous activity should be avoided for one month—no weight-bearing machines at the gym—as they can temporarily elevate the blood pressure and result in hemorrhage under the facial skin. No sex for the first week to 10 days. Let your surgeon tell you when and what you can do to resume your normal athletic routine. Many patients can expect to return to work within two weeks. Remember: The healing process will continue internally for several more months.

The best, fully realized results may not be apparent for several months or up to a year. After two weeks, however, you'll see improvement nearly every day until the neck and lower face normalize. Final results may take at least nine months to a year.

Possible complications:

Complications tend to be rare with this procedure, although infection and hematomas (as with all surgeries) are possibilities. Portions of the chin may feel numb and, in varying degrees, the numbness may

Watch Out!
One troublesome complication that may follow fat removal through an incision under the chin is adherence of the incision to the underlying muscle. This produces a noticeable depression. This problem is usually related to overzealous excision of fat and can usually be prevented by leaving a small amount of fat attached to the undersurface of the skin.

continue for up to nine months or a year, when final results can be assessed.

With men, surgically removing too much skin can cause tightly sutured wounds to be pulled; this may be due to excising more skin than appropriate. All patients should be aware of this potential result that tends to yield an abnormally wide scar, which can often be camouflaged with make-up. In severe cases, scar revision may be necessary. But eradicating or diminishing the scar may not be a realistic expectation. However, in order to remove the gobbler, many patients are quite willing to tolerate the scar formation.

The weekend lift

This is an evolving, controversial procedure that has been developed and introduced by dermatologist William Cook, MD, of Coronado, California. The procedure's true point of difference is the use of a laser inside the neck, on the flaccid tissue that contributes to a jowly look. Featured as part of ABC's investigative *20/20* television program, the procedure was promoted as the "Weekend Alternative to a Face Lift." This is a bit of an overstatement, since only the area below the jaw line is treated. Nasolabial folds, facial wrinkles, and deep furrows that are above the jaw line are not remedied.

The genesis of an idea

For prospects who have lost jaw definition due to a double chin, the weekend lift procedure can provide dramatic results, and these results do contribute to a younger-looking face. Dr. Cook has performed nearly 500 operations with his unique procedure. He has lectured extensively to thousands of doctors in the U.S. and abroad and personally trained 25 other doctors in the intricacies of his approach.

The inspiration for Dr. Cook's innovation came from his interest and expertise in treating skin conditions with the ultrapulsed laser. Results were typically excellent, but he was very much aware of two considerable healing downsides of traditional laser treatment that troubled patients who had to return to the office within two weeks or so:

- Weeks of raw, tender skin that is quite noticeable

- The extreme pinkness or redness that prevails for months in some cases

He wondered if the laser, used inside on exposed tissue, could cause the same tightening without the outside facial skin enduring the long and uncomfortable healing of a traditional laser treatment. The laser is used after the area's fat is removed by liposuction. According to Dr. Cook, with the tightening comes the laying down of new collagen and elastic fibers that make the surface new, supple, and rejuvenated. But when done on the inside, the healing takes place beneath the outside skin layer.

The procedure's point of difference

The laser works a bit like a vacuum food sealer that removes unwanted air pockets. Following the liposuctioning of fat, the laser takes a loose, flaccid area and gives it tone as the treated section shrinks. Picture, if you will, a strip of thin, raw chicken breast, skinned. Supple and fleshy before heat or a flame is applied, it tightens and contracts as it cooks. In the process, the flesh becomes more firm and appears more dense.

Here are the details on Dr. Cook's innovative procedure.

Common name: Dr. Cook's weekend lift
What it does: Removes excess chin fat via liposuction and tightens the flaccid underlying tissue by laser application inside the neck
Price range: $6,000 to $12,000
Operation duration: One and a half hours or less
Anesthetic: Local or local with sedation (MAC)
The procedure:
After the patient is sedated, the patient's skin is cleaned and marked with a surgical pen. Pockets of fat are circled and the outline of new contours is sketched in. The neck area is then injected with a tumescent anesthetic. Lidocaine further numbs the area and epinephrine causes the vessels to constrict. Because the skin puffs up and away from the underlying tissue, bruising is virtually eliminated. Dr. Cook follows the typical steps for liposuctioning fatty deposits in the neck after he uses the laser to cut an incision which runs lengthwise under the chin. If possible, Dr. Cook will frequently camouflage the incision in a natural fold.

After removing the fat (and using this opening), the doctor slips the laser beneath the subcutaneous layer and heats or zaps portions of the flaccid tissue, causing the underside to shrink and tighten. As in other (albeit less controversial) neck rejuvenating procedures, the doctor then stitches the neck muscles or adds a chin implant for greater definition. Excess skin is removed and the incision is sutured closed.

Postoperative expectations:
The treated area is girdled with strips of a thin, foam protective tape. In some cases, it appears as if the patient is wearing a helmet, though the protective gear is much like that worn following any other face-lift or neck-lift procedure. The procedure is called

the weekend alternative to a face lift because many patients schedule surgery on Friday morning. Then, on the following Monday, the tape is gently removed and only mild swelling or minor bruising is likely to be present. Mild pain or a tight discomfort has been reported. Sutures to close the incision are removed on the Monday following surgery or shortly thereafter.

Possible complications:

Remember that this is a controversial approach that has not been proven over time, and there are many plastic surgeons who challenge the average dermatologist's ability to perform surgery. Because it is new, the long-term effects are not known. Dr. Cook claims there are no serious postoperative complications related to this procedure. However, many surgeons question the use of a laser inside the neck, viewing the approach as too radical to correct healthy, living tissue. Also, the procedure is not yet recognized by the leading plastic surgery boards and societies.

Just the facts

- Neck contours and skin conditions vary widely; seek the appropriate correction for your desired results.

- Seeking neck modification earlier rather than later may result in a less invasive procedure.

- A chin implant may also help create a better overall facial contour and a more pleasing, youthful result.

- If the neck requires major skin and fat removal to restore tone, the patient may require an incision that produces a more noticeable scar.

Reshaping Facial Features

PART IV

GET THE SCOOP ON...
Common eye corrections ▪ Why nose jobs
create the highest patient dissatisfaction ▪
Understanding nose dynamics to ensure a
better result ▪ Correcting common adult ear
and earlobe problems

Procedures for Eyes, Nose, and Ears

There's a famous quote attributed to the turn-of-the-century financial wizard, J. P. Morgan. When asked how much his yacht cost, he replied, "If you have to ask, you can't afford one." Despite his fantastic wealth, J. P. couldn't buy a normal nose. He suffered from rosacea, a skin disorder in which broken blood vessels covered his large, bulbous nose. In fact, one hostess of the day, perhaps overwhelmed by Morgan's proboscis, asked, as a tea cup was passed, "Mr. Morgan, one or two cubes of sugar with your nose?"

I imagine if medicine offered then what it offers prospects today, Mr. Morgan probably would have bought his own state-of-the-art hospital and surgical team. Cyrano de Bergerac, on the other hand—or so I imagine—would not change; as a gallant, sensitive lover, he claimed, "A great nose indicates a great man—genial, courteous, intellectual, virile, courageous."

The eyes, nose, and ears play an important role in establishing a person's character. Our features truly define who we are. In this chapter, you'll see how several minor operations—some making only very small changes—can add balance to the face. Some operations are practically over before you get comfortable in the surgeon's seat! So if you're considering changing an aspect of your eyes, nose, or ears, read on.

Eye procedures that freshen your look

One type of lower lid surgery typically requires no suturing following the excision.

Common name: pouch removal, eye-bag job (subconjunctival blepharoplasty)

What it does: Removes puffiness and bags from the lower lid

Price range: $1,500 to $4,000

Operation duration: About an hour

Anesthetic: Local or local with sedation (MAC)

The procedure:

This is a rapid-healing procedure that requires a small incision but, in many cases, no sutures. If sutures are used, they are the kind that dissolve. This operation is often used to treat young adults who have a pouchy look below the lower lid (see the following before and after photos). Most prospects

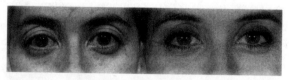

Puffy lower lids (left) give a fatigued appearance to any youthful person. The photo on the right shows correction to both upper and lower lids. (Source: Dr. Gregory LaTrenta)

appear fatigued and tired even after a restful vacation. Typically this puffy appearance is hereditary.

Sometimes the puffiness crops up in college years and many prospects incorrectly feel that once their intensive study routine slows down and they resume a more normal life, the puffiness will dissipate. Unfortunately, most of us can't leave undesirable genetic tendencies on campus when we hit the job market.

To reduce the patient's tired, weary appearance, the surgeon pulls down on the lower lid (with the cornea protected), makes an incision in the soft, moist eyelid lining, called the conjunctiva, and removes the pockets of fat.

After the fat is removed, the surgeon applies ointment and returns the eyelid to its normal position. Some surgeons prefer to repair the incision with absorbable sutures.

If the prospect's skin is flaccid, this procedure is not recommended. The best candidates have elastic, toned skin that will tighten to give a refreshed and smooth appearance, making the eyes appear less wan.

Postoperative expectations:

Healing (with or without sutures) is speedy, and some bruising may be evident. Patients who diligently follow their surgeon's recommended protocol, drink plenty of fluids, and follow a healthy lifestyle are amazed at the significant improvement this fairly simple procedure delivers. Smokers and heavy drinkers, unsurprisingly, may compromise results, meaning their puffiness and swelling may return more quickly. How long the results last varies with each patient; though an average of five or more years can be expected.

Unofficially...
In many blepharoplasty procedures, pockets of fat are removed with forceps that are so fine, one could dip into a bowl of Caspian caviar and remove a single, practically microscopic, precious black pearl.

Possible complications:

There are few complications to this procedure, though contact lens wearers must avoid pulling on the lower lid to insert contacts. In rare cases, infection has occurred but is usually remedied with a prescription for antibiotics. If your eyes had any asymmetry to begin with, the procedure may accent this unevenness, though most surgeons with great aesthetic vision will compensate for this during the procedure.

Common name: rounding the Eastern or Asian eye

What it does: Diminishes the almond-shaped characteristic of the Asian eye

Price range: $2,000 to $5,000

Operation duration: Under two hours

Anesthetic: Local

The procedure:

This procedure can make an Eastern eye appear more rounded. Because the operation diminishes an ethnic characteristic, it is often decried as a useless procedure for Asians. The procedure, however, does not remove evidence of a person's racial heritage. Though the patient is sedated, frequently the patient's eyes remain open during the surgery. This permits the careful surgeon to observe each individual's symmetry. As the balance is checked throughout the operation, the surgeon essentially creates a fold in the upper lid. This crease is absent in most Asian people.

An incision is made in each of the upper eyelids. Skin, muscle, and sometimes fatty tissue are excised. Temporary or permanent stitches may be sewn into the underlying muscle to anchor its position during healing and temporary stitches are also placed in the skin. Some doctors stitch the skin to the levator muscle which rests inside the eyelid.

Postoperative expectations:

To minimize postoperative swelling and discoloration, iced compresses must be applied continuously for 24 hours for optimum results. The patient rests with the head elevated to further minimize swelling of the eyelids. Periodically, ointment may be placed in the eyes and over the incision lines to protect the eye and minimize crusting of the suture line.

There is rarely pain, but do expect some discomfort. Severe eye pain suggests the possibility of a complication—call your surgeon immediately if this occurs. Most patients experience tightness for several weeks as the sutures heal and tighten. If the operation was performed in a hospital, the patient is usually discharged on the day of the surgery with instructions to continue applying iced compresses. Ointment is applied to the suture lines three or four times a day and placed in the eye at night. If the eyes are dry, artificial tears are used as often as necessary. At the time of discharge, the patient frequently has swollen eyelids; discoloration follows shortly thereafter. Much of this bruising disappears in seven to ten days but may linger longer. In some cases, there is virtually no bruising and very little swelling.

You should be able to close your eye shortly after the surgery, though it will feel very tender.

Possible complications:

Risks include infection and the formation of hematomas, though the incidence of either for this surgery tends to be very low. A surgeon with a good deal of experience in performing this ethnic modification should be able to outline any special individual considerations prior to the surgery. Any sharp pain, frequently an indication of a serious

Watch Out!
Some patients have reported a temporary blurring of vision which may linger for several days. This, too, can be minimized by keeping the eye moist with artificial tears. Occasionally other types of eye drops may be necessary; consult with your surgeon on this.

problem, must be reported to your surgeon immediately. It is crucial to find an experienced surgeon
who can anticipate any aesthetic variables of asymmetry inherent to each patient's face, in order to
deliver highly even, desirable aesthetic results.

Common name: minor laser or lower-lid clamp

What it does: Removes excess, crinkled sun-damaged
skin that appears in the lower eyelid area

Price range: $1,000 to $2,000

Operation duration: Less than an hour

Anesthetic: Local

The procedure:

Bright Idea
The clamping
procedure can
also be used as a
minor touch-up
on someone who
has had an eye
job several or
more years ago
and wishes to
remove small
amounts of
loose skin.

Frequently, young adults (or some middle-age
prospects) with sun damage near the outer corner
of the lower lid can benefit from clamping, a reasonably simple procedure that removes the excess
crepe and loose skin that remains crinkled. With the
clamp procedure, the small folds can be locally anesthetized and gently lifted with an instrument much
like a tweezers that clamps rather than plucks. As
the skin is compressed, fine scissors remove the
excess, and simple sutures remain in place for two
or three days. Minor laser resurfacing can also
remove these extra folds that appear in those people
who spend a great deal of time in the sun, such as
avid skiers and tennis buffs. There is virtually no
bleeding, swelling, or significant discomfort with
laser resurfacing.

Postoperative expectations:

Because there is very little trauma to the area, most
patients breeze through the quick procedure without much, if any, bruising. Vigilant application of ice
compresses can practically eradicate any swelling.
There is virtually no pain, but it's likely most
patients will feel an unusual tightness in the treated

area. If done on a Friday, sutures can be removed on Monday and you may be back at work that day—or shortly thereafter—without any hint of having had the surgery.

Possible complications:

Because the procedure is a minor one, there are few complications, although removing too much skin can create an unnatural look.

Reshaping the nose

Nose resculpting, though it's been around for many decades, requires incredible ability by the surgeon. Many of the top surgeons in their field spent years seeking to master this highly individualized and demanding procedure. How did many of them learn? Dr. Stephen Grifka, a leading plastic surgeon in Culver City, California, explains, "During procedures, my teachers placed my hand on top of theirs. It's a way to experience the shaping and feel the dynamics of what is, essentially, a blind, unseen operation." We Americans have a much higher incidence of nose jobs than most other countries. Most Europeans find this trend appalling. To them, the profile declares one's pedigree. Some Italians claim to be able to decipher the intricacies of a family tree (and where a person's family roots can be traced within a hundred mile radius) by studying their compatriot's nose.

But if you decide you want to reshape your nose, here are the most common procedures.

Common name: nose job, nose resculpting (rhinoplasty)

What it does: Alters the nose's shape and size to create a different profile and bring facial features into balance

Price range: $3,000 to $9,000
Operation duration: Usually under two hours
Anesthetic: General or local with sedation (MAC)
The procedure:

Most nose surgeries are performed through incisions made on the inside of the nose; though in some cases, small outside incisions are used to reduce the width and flare of the nostrils. The latter approach is considered by many surgeons to be a last resort—when no other option will yield the aesthetic results that both the patient and surgeon seek. In the best-case scenario, these outside scars usually fade to become imperceptible after healing. However, it is not uncommon for scars to be visible and remain so for a long time. Since the nose is a key facial feature and a prominent one, you must study with great scrutiny a doctor's photos of patients before and after surgery. Talk to former patients who have had outside (nostril) work.

In many typical cases, after the anesthetic is administered, the surgeon also applies—inside of the nose—gauze dipped in extra numbing medication. Many surgeons call rhinoplasty the blind procedure, meaning that the delicate touch of the surgeon's hands shapes what the eye cannot see. What forms the nose, apart from skin and tissue, is the placement and shape of nasal bone material and nasal cartilage.

Use your fingers to take a short tour of your nose so you can see how it's configured. Start at the top and place your fingers between your brow area. Now drop down a notch and touch the *frontal bone.* It's found before the nose begins to protrude and is the foundation for two *nasal bones* that create a rooflike shape that extends out, forming on each side the *maxillary bone,* which travels downward to the flexible lower two-thirds of the *nasal skeleton,* which consists of cartilage.

The skin over the nose tends to be of varying thickness; often thinning toward the middle and becoming sturdier, even thicker at the nasal root, which is the junction where the forehead meets the nose. (That's the area that most bosses pinch, squinting their eyes shut, when an employee asks for a raise at the end of the day.) The lower part of the nose is usually blessed with lots of oil glands, making it the most powdered female facial feature.

Inside the nose, approached from either side of the nostril, incisions are made and the nose skin is elevated from the underlying bone and cartilage. Using specially designed instruments—some are like small sculpting chisels—the surgeon modifies the nasal skeleton. The hump of the bridge, called the dorsal bone, may be reduced by filing. More significant reshaping of the bone may require making careful and precise fractures that produce postoperative swelling and significant bruising. This breaking or fracturing process is the key reason for the blackened eyes that occur after rhinoplasty. Wide bones that are fractured are then repositioned to achieve the desired contour. Finally, the alar cartilage, which produces each nostril's flaring arch ridge, is sculpted to refine the nose tip. The incisions are closed with dissolving sutures. Any nasal packing used earlier to deliver a numbing anesthetic to the lining is removed. This packing also tends to constrict blood vessels and control nasal bleeding, which can be quite intense.

Fresh packing is inserted to hold the septum in place during healing. The spongy septum has an enduring memory and will do practically anything to return to its original preoperative shape; the packing, like a strict 19th-century posture brace, discourages this. An external dressing and splint minimize dripping and movement. Together they act to brace the sensitive area.

Postoperative expectations:

The range of how quickly each patient bounces back varies considerably. For some, the pain is slight. For others, breathing is stuffy for a long while, though they may have endured little or no other discomfort. Others have throbbing pain but, thanks to medication, can rest comfortably, sleeping for most of the first, even second day.

Nearly all patients share one obvious distinction: A not-very-discreet dressing remains on the nose for a week to 10 days.

Cold, dry compresses are generally applied at frequent intervals for the first 24 hours to minimize bruising and swelling. And you may feel true, unequivocal pain. In most cases, your nose has been broken!

After 24 hours, mildly warm compresses can help diminish bruising and swelling. Some patients prefer to continue cold compresses during this time; others prefer warm compresses. Be sure to follow your doctor's specific protocol.

You may swallow some blood in the course of the operation. Don't be alarmed if your stool darkens before returning to normal. A mild, simple liquid diet is best to start your recovery. Take small sips of any healthy clear liquid, such as water, juice, or clear soups—no carbonated sodas (you don't want bubbles in your nose!). Be sure that your stomach is settled before resuming normal eating and drinking.

Bright Idea
During recovery from nose surgery, you can breathe through your mouth only. Keep plenty of liquids close by. It's also a good idea to sleep in a room with a humidifier.

Nausea and vomiting can complicate your healing; notify your doctor immediately.

Expect two black, swollen eyes. You may or may not get them, but if you do, you'll be better prepared to live with them for a week to 10 days, until the bruising subsides. Contact lenses can't be worn, but you may find it tolerable—though just barely—to tape your eyeglasses to your forehead for the first week. It will be somewhat gentler than resting them on the bridge of your nose.

Follow your surgeon's protocol on showering, though most feel it's okay as long as you keep the splint dry.

The tape and bandage are removed five to ten days after the procedure, along with any packing. (The latter may be removed prior to the bandage.) The nose is still swollen at this time and not a good representation of final results.

Be aware that minor changes evolve over the ensuing 18 months as scar tissue matures. Final results are not entirely evident for a good year, as seen in the following photos.

Unofficially...
Although 90 percent of nose swelling usually diminishes by the end of the second postoperative week, the remaining 10 percent subsides very slowly. Final (or near-final) results may take six months or more.

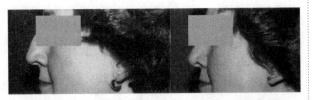

A reduction in the overall size of the nose brings an attractive harmony to the face, as does the modification to the bridge. (Source: Dr. Stephen Grifka)

Care must be taken to prevent injury during the postoperative period; swelling and even an undesirable shifting or movement of the fragile bones can occur.

Exposure to the sun should be avoided for at least six months to prevent increased pigmentation of the nasal skin. However, most surgeons don't balk at sunbathing one month after surgery as long as you use a heavy-duty, effective sunscreen.

Possible complications:

Nose surgery can present the highest level of patient dissatisfaction. It requires significant expertise on the surgeon's part. The surgery is demanding because, as surgeons describe the operation, it is a blind surgery. Since many variables affect the final outcome, complications, too, vary. Perhaps the most common complication is the development of fullness in the area just above the nasal tip. This fullness is frequently related to accumulation of scar tissue. Called a polly beak or parrot's beak, because of the appearance of the nasal profile, this problem is more common to large noses and noses with thick skin. In some cases, this deformity is accentuated by a gradual settling of the tip. If detected early, many polly beaks can be eliminated by a series of cortisone-type injections effective in reducing scar tissue. Polly beaks that do not respond to cortisone—or those due to other things besides excessive scar tissue—are treated by revision surgery. But be forewarned! Subsequent procedures have limitations and the possibility to improve a contour or get what you hoped for diminishes with each subsequent correction. Corrective surgery should be delayed until at least a year following the primary procedure.

Excessive removal of nasal bone may produce a ski jump or Bob Hope-like profile; most procedures done in the early '70s seemed to deliver an undesirable one-size–fits-all look. As surgeons learned more and gained technical expertise, this ski nose result declined somewhat. (Cosmetic ways to modify the ski nose result are explained in the next procedure.) When a long nose is shortened and pulled up" to its new position, any excessive shortening can result in a pig snout, which is to be avoided in all cases. Excessive removal of the nasal tip cartilage may produce irregularities or pinching of the tip and require extensive surgery to correct.

On occasion, a small residual nasal hump in the bridge area may appear after swelling is resolved. This is more common after removal of a large hump, or in a nose with thick skin. If this hump is objectionable, it can easily be corrected with a revision operation.

Bleeding may occur in the early postoperative period and is managed like an ordinary bloody nose: tilt the head back, place a tissue or gauze pad under each nostril, and remain still. If bleeding persists, call your doctor and don't panic. In some cases, nasal packing may have to be reinserted.

Nasal obstruction sometimes occurs after nasal surgery. Temporary breathing difficulty during the early postoperative period may be due to swelling or the result of an upper respiratory infection or allergy. Persistent nasal obstruction may be a consequence of a septal deviation or abnormality of the turbinates—the underlying nasal cavity bones covered with mucous membranes. Often referred to as a "stuffy nose" or a sinus problem, this condition may require further treatment.

Infection, noted by a mild rise in temperature, is a rare complication of rhinoplasty, but it can be extremely harmful and ravaging if it occurs. Infection is more common if the surgery is performed while the patient has a cold or is

Moneysaver
Some surgeons routinely remove septal deviations during rhinoplasty on the assumption that these areas may become symptomatic after the size of the nose is reduced. If you have any current breathing problems, treating a septum problem might be covered by your medical insurance. Check with your carrier first.

experiencing a major allergic reaction. If you fear an infection is underway—you have an unusual nasal discharge or experience considerable pain and unusual swelling—contact your surgeon immediately.

Common name: athletic nose or French bridge, nasal implant

What it does: Provides a natural, pleasing ridge or hump to a flat nose; corrects rhinoplasties that result in a ski nose

Price range: $3,000 to $9,000

Operation duration: Varies, but usually under two hours

Anesthetic: Local with sedation (MAC)

The procedure:

Since nose resculpting has the highest percentage of patient dissatisfaction as well as a considerable incidence of aesthetic complications, secondary surgery—or follow-up procedures—are more common after this surgery than other cosmetic surgeries. Nasal implants are often necessary to make the correction. Implants may be made from bone, cartilage, or synthetic materials. Apart from modifying previous operations, nasal implants are also used to modify hereditary traits, such as a broad or flat nose.

Postoperative expectations:

Like most rhinoplasty operations, cold compresses must be applied continuously to the nose and eyes for 24 hours to minimize swelling and discoloration. Following protocol can seriously reduce postoperative bruising and swelling that is so endemic to this particular procedure. You should expect to stay in bed, propping your head on fluffy pillows to keep the nose and area elevated to further minimize swelling. The degree of swelling and discoloration varies, depending to a large extent on the thickness of the patient's bone and nasal skin as well as his normal healing ability.

Possible complications:
Most implant procedures that are not performed as follow-up, corrective surgeries deliver satisfactory to excellent results with few if any complications. In some cases, the implant can become loose, but this is typically traceable to a physical injury that occurs after the surgery and is not due to day-to-day normal activities. If the procedure is a corrective surgery, the patient must expect limited results. With each successive correction, the chance for major improvement diminishes.

Procedures for the ears

Small ears, even the most perfect shapes that rest flat against the head, rarely turn anyone's head. The most perfect ears may resemble delicate seashells, but few people will ever remark on their aesthetic appeal. However, ears that visibly protrude seem to draw the eye. Many people dismiss the ear as a silly aesthetic beacon, but those who have protruding ears may simply want to look into the mirror and not see their ears.

Common name: ear job (otoplasty)

What it does: Places protruding ears closer to the face, corrects imbalances, and restores facial harmony

Price range: $1,500 per ear or $2,000 or more for both, depending on ear configuration and health of cartilage

Operation duration: About an hour or more per ear

Anesthetic: General or local with sedation (MAC)

The procedure:

Ears tend to have a normal crease in the cartilage that rolls the outer rim forward, placing the outside rim somewhat close to the head. In jug ears, this cartilage—called the antihelix—unfurls much like a flag that flaps backward. Another anatomical variable, an abundance of cartilage, can create the appearance of disproportionately large ears.

Seeking medical attention at the time of an outer ear injury is ideal. Many simply do not view an ear injury as serious enough and even early intervention may not be sufficient to restore the ear's appearance. With ears, surgical repair is possible at any age.

In cosmetic ear surgery, the doctor seeks to re-create the natural anatomical folds of the cartilage. This may or may not involve removal of cartilage, but it almost always involves carving and suturing the cartilage.

An incision is made on the back of the ear to expose the cartilage so that it can be sculpted or folded. Occasionally, a piece of cartilage will be removed to provide a more natural-looking fold. Sutures are used to fold the cartilage back on itself to reshape the ear; permanent sutures may be used to hold the integrity of the new shape. In some cases, excess skin is removed if ear reduction is necessary. Variations on this basic procedure can effectively modify and correct a wide variety of external-ear deformities.

Postoperative expectations:

The patient frequently experiences throbbing pain of moderate intensity during the first 24 hours. For some, outer ear pain prevents a good night's rest for the first week or so. Others seem to experience little discomfort, unless the ear is touched, even gently.

Watch Out!
Damage to the ear cartilage occurs more frequently in athletes who assiduously pursue contact sports. Many weekend sports enthusiasts are surprised to learn that ear damage and bleeding effectively damage cartilage, causing the outer ear to become knotted and gnarled—hence the proverbial cauliflower ear sometimes seen on professional fighters.

Bed rest and elevation of the head minimize general postoperative discomfort, and pain-relieving medications are prescribed as needed.

The dressing is removed the day after surgery and the ears are carefully examined for signs of bleeding or accumulation of blood beneath the skin surface. If a hematoma is found, it will be promptly drained. For the most part, the ears are considerably swollen, discolored, and tender. The dressing is reapplied and left in place for four to seven days unless the patient complains of increasing pain, which suggests development of a hematoma or infection. The sutures are removed in five to seven days, though some surgeons prefer absorbable stitches.

Although most of the discoloration has disappeared when the dressing is removed, the ear will remain tender and somewhat swollen for several weeks.

Injury during this period causes considerable pain and may contribute to bleeding or infection, so alert your surgeon to any injury, however slight.

Possible complications:

Significant complications rarely occur after otoplasty. The most common postoperative problem relates to bleeding, though reopening the incision is unusual. If hematomas are not removed, they may cause cartilage damage and infection. Small hematomas can frequently be removed with a needle; larger ones may require making an incision over their pooling surface.

Infection rarely follows otoplasty, but its occurrence can be devastating if it spreads into the very vulnerable cartilage. For this reason the ear must be carefully inspected any time you sense an increase in pain in the early postoperative period. Any slight indication must be brought to your surgeon's

Bright Idea
In order to protect the area during healing, your surgeon will likely recommend a soft, not-too-tight tennis or ski headband to substitute for a bandage. During the first week the band can be worn constantly. For about three weeks thereafter, the band, worn while sleeping or moving around, will protect the ear.

attention immediately. Redness of the ear, particularly around the incision, and low-grade fever are common signs of infection. Antibiotics and draining of localized areas of pus generally resolve infection. Without treatment, the infected ear can be ravaged hideously, leaving little healthy cartilage to work with for any secondary procedure.

Excessive scar tissue around the incision occasionally follows otoplasty, but the exact reasons for this remain unclear. Hypertrophied scarring, a result of the skin being stretched too much to comfortably bear the stress and pull of the sutures, is more common in dark-skinned people. In many cases these scars gradually mature and fade spontaneously. In others, injection of cortisone into the scar may help reduce the ridge. Occasionally scar excision can minimize this reaction.

The possibility of the ear protruding again must be carefully discussed with the patient before the surgery; it's a risk inherent to the procedure. A second operation may be necessary to reposition the ear or to correct asymmetry.

Overcorrecting of prominent ears can result in a too flat, plastered-down appearance—a result top ear surgeons criticize as glued-down and unnatural looking. Not so if you ask the patients. Most don't care a whit about this flat look. To them, it's a terrifically happy reversal of their former appearance.

Common name: keloid surgery

What it does: Removes a balloon-like collection of scar tissue that may form on the earlobe

Price range: $500, more if the repair requires a complicated reconstruction

Duration: Usually less than an hour

Anesthetic: Local

The procedure:

A typical keloid, usually called a keloid scar, is an odd-shaped tissue that seems to be covered with a taut, smooth, balloonlike skin.

Most keloids hang from the earlobe, but others may appear on the chin or other facial area. The keloid is treated by excision and the area is closed with sutures; often these are dissolving sutures. Keloids on the ear are often traceable to a normal, uncomplicated ear piercing. Keloids result from a healing scar that automatically keeps producing extra tissue. Young African-American adults often show a higher incidence of keloids.

Keloids are not cancerous and simply result from a genetic predisposition toward uncontrolled scarring. After a wound has healed and repaired itself, the body forgets to shut off scar formation. Some keloids can be difficult to permanently eliminate because the same genetic trigger (however poorly understood) that initially created keloids continues despite the removal. Nevertheless, nearly all keloids can be removed surgically; many are discouraged from recurring with steroid injections. Some doctors prescribe a very low-dose, targeted X-ray treatment that ceases keloid production in the treated area.

The important consideration is to understand that keloids are not life-threatening; however, their removal can instantly enhance a person's appearance and feeling of well-being.

Postoperative expectations:

An antibiotic ointment may be prescribed, and the area must be kept clean and sterile; pull hair away from the site until healing is complete. To reduce pain or swelling, apply ice compresses as directed by

Unofficially...
Most ear keloids range wildly in size; some are as small as a pearl, while others can be as large as— or even larger than—a Ping-Pong ball!

your doctor for the first night and day following the surgery. For most patients, the pain is quite minimal and about as tough to bear as an ear piercing. After the first 24 hours, there is little discomfort. Each patient must be vigilant about hygiene; infection will follow if strict protocol is not followed. Sutures are either dissolve or can be removed by the nurse or doctor, usually three to five days after surgery.

Possible complications:

Complications are not likely, but infection can compromise healing. Keep the suture area sterile. Your doctor will determine if antibiotic ointment or another medication is necessary. In the past, if you experienced itching from internal lobe bumps—these too are keloids—you may also have some of this same irritation after surgery. In most cases, these bumps will dissolve on their own. As mentioned, not all keloids successfully disappear following excision; they may reappear.

Common name: earlobe repair

What it does: Corrects torn earlobe rims

Price range: $300

Operation duration: Less than 45 minutes

Anesthetic: Local

The procedure:

It's fairly ordinary for people with pierced ears to experience stretched earlobe holes. It can be due to heavy earrings, or the lobe itself may thin over time. When earrings are heavy, apart from causing drooped holes, they may stretch the earlobes, which may become pendulous, imparting an older look to the face. In some people, the earlobe hole is stretched so much that it no longer supports a post-type earring. Accidental tearing or catching the earring may cause the jewelry to rip completely through the lobe, leaving a bifid, or forked, earlobe. Using local anesthetic, the surgeon excises the torn rim and sews the edges together. Sutures are usually removed in seven to ten days, and the resulting scar looks like a natural crease in the earlobe.

Postoperative expectations:

The ear is protected by soft cotton pads soaked in glycerin or mineral oil to cradle the area and permit the patient to rest as comfortably as possible.

For most patients, the pain is quite minimal. After the first 24 hours, there is little discomfort, though applying cold compresses following the surgery helps reduce any pain and swelling. Antibiotics may be given, and keeping the area sterile and clean is essential for healthy healing. Usually, after six to eight weeks, the ear can be repierced in a different area.

Possible complications:

Complications are rare, though any prospect who has suffered from the formation of small, internal earlobe bumps may experience some of this same irritation. In most cases, these irregularities will dissolve on their own.

Watch Out!
If you choose to repierce your ear, be sure to avoid the new scar completely. It isn't strong enough—nor will it ever be—to support earrings.

Common name: earlobe reduction or augmentation

What it does: Reshapes each earlobe

Price range: $500 to $800 per lobe

Operation duration: An hour or less

Anesthetic: Local

The procedure:

Some prospects note a progressive enlargement of the earlobes, which become long and floppy and makes wearing earrings difficult. A reduction is done in a manner similar to earlobe repair. The back of the lobe may be the key site because suturing there can hide the scar.

For thinning lobes, fat grafts taken from the patient (from areas such as the buttocks) can add bulk to the lobes and are usually placed through incisions in the back of the lobe. Grafts are small and transferred with their own blood supply that helps regenerate a healthy regrowth of appropriate bulk.

Postoperative expectations:

In some cases, the ear is protected by soft cotton pads soaked in glycerin or mineral oil. The pads cradle the area and help the patient to rest as comfortably as possible.

For most patients, depending on how much of the lobe has been treated, the pain is typically quite minimal. After the first 24 hours, there is little pronounced discomfort; some patients report a mild throbbing sensation, which is normal. Cold compresses applied after the surgery help reduce pain and swelling. Antibiotics may be given, and keeping the area sterile and clean is essential for healthy healing. Usually, after six to eight weeks, revisions can be done if necessary.

Postoperative complications:

Complications are rare and not likely, though keeping the area clear of debris or unclean material is crucial. Also, some prospects who have suffered from the formation of small, internal earlobe bumps may experience some of this same irritation. In most cases, these irregularities will resolve on their own.

Just the facts

- Since eyes are a key expressive feature, corrective cosmetic procedures to the upper or lower lids usually delivers a greater harmony to the person's appearance.

- Nose surgery has the highest percentage of patient dissatisfaction; even though the procedure may appear commonplace, seek the most qualified surgeon you can find.

- Understand the risks of nose surgery, including the possible loss of clear breathing and sinus problems thereafter.

- Don't proceed with nose surgery unless you have a clear understanding of how corrective, or secondary surgery, may also compromise results.

- Poor hygiene can contribute to infection or compromise aesthetic results.

GET THE SCOOP ON...
The dynamics and types of implants ▪ How the
chin provides facial harmony ▪ Innovations for
the lips ▪ The role of collagen and fat injections

Chapter 11

Recontouring the Face: Cheeks, Chin, and Lips

Many surgeons stress that small cosmetic changes can deliver big results. There is a great deal of truth to this, especially within the realm of implants. These augmenting devices, mostly synthetic, can enlarge a receding chin to impart a totally new profile. Other applications, such as adding height or roundness to cheeks, can make a person appear more rested and alert. Your mouth, one of the more expressive features you have, can also be enhanced to give a plumper, fuller look.

Apart from facial implants, many cosmetic doctors still prefer collagen injections. Other doctors swear that a patient's own fat is the best source for plumping a mild fold or crease. In this chapter we'll explore the dynamics of each method and its potential limitations so you can make a wise choice. Here's what you need to know to determine whether the cost, time, and recovery are worth the result you seek.

Sculpting and reshaping facial features

The development of implants that are easily shaped and molded created a surge in cosmetic applications. Some patients rushed to have their wrinkles plumped up, others sought to even out their cheekbones, jaw, or chin. Unlike injectable liquid fillers, most of these man-made implants are permanent; many are pliant and as reasonably soft as the human tissue they seek to replicate.

Implant material can also be harvested from your own soft tissue, called *fascia*. Fascia is a strong connective tissue that covers muscles and connects them to one another and to other structures. Common anatomical donor fascia includes thigh or temple fascia. Other materials useful for implant are bone from hip or skull area and nose or ear cartilage.

These implant materials have the capability of becoming part of the living tissue in the transplanted area or, if unsuccessful, they may be partially or even fully absorbed by the body with no attendant problems.

Many cosmetic augmentations are done with synthetic implants. Because they are biologically inert, implants remain unchanged. However, the body may respond to the implanted material by forming a scar that cradles the implant, which may distort the correction. Synthetic implants may also become extruded or cause late infection.

Synthetic facial implants are generally used to add balance or create heft. Each procedure is customized to every patient's needs. Measurements are taken preoperatively and an appropriately sized implant is chosen. Be sure you and your surgeon discuss varying sizes and shapes during the preliminary consultation; ask to see a sample of the proposed implant.

Unofficially...
Bone implants are used to reconstruct large segments of missing facial bone. This is based on the surgical guideline that, whenever possible, tissue is replaced with like tissue.

As a rule, implants are placed during outpatient procedures, and many facial implants can be placed using local anesthetic alone. It is common, however, to use local anesthetic with sedation. Complex procedures require use of a general anesthetic, invariably those that relate to significant chin surgery. For facial implants—chin, jaw, and sometimes cheek areas—many incisions are placed inside the mouth. If external incisions are used, they are typically in the lower eyelid for cheek implants and in the crease under the chin for chin implants.

Prescription pain medication will be needed for the first three to five days. Over-the-counter analgesics may be indicated for one to two weeks.

Severe pain may be indicative of problems. You should be aware of risks that specifically relate to implants, including:

- Bleeding around an implant may cause a medical emergency known as *compartment syndrome*. This condition, if not addressed immediately, may halt circulation to nerves and muscles in the area, causing them to weaken, shrink, and stop functioning. Ask your doctor about symptoms in the specific area that may signal this bleeding.

- An implant may become dislodged. Usually this is caused by physical trauma to the area. A second operation may be required to reposition the implant.

- Pressure caused by the presence of the implant may erode the underlying bone. This is a late occurrence that may happen over many years, but it almost always occurs to some degree even though it may not cause a problem for most people.

In most cases, augments are readily accepted by the body. Most fluid or blood accumulation around the implant resolves itself spontaneously or requires mild surgical drainage. Infection around an implant should be treated with antibiotics. If an infection persists, the implant must usually be removed.

During the first week following the procedure, you will need to keep your head elevated at all times when you sleep to minimize bruising and swelling. A recliner chair or several firm pillows will keep you in the proper position.

The area around any implant will be bruised and swollen for seven to ten days. If you've had sutures placed inside your mouth, perfect oral hygiene is critically important. Follow your doctor's recommended protocol precisely!

Within a week, the stitches inside your mouth will dissolve and should vanish within 10 days. Antibiotics, as a preventative measure, are usually prescribed for up to 10 days.

Many of the more popular facial procedures that reshape the face rely on the use of implants. Here are the more popular ways to augment your face and make other cosmetic changes.

Plumping cheeks

Within the world of cosmetics, Americans spend millions of dollars for bronzers and cheek blush. Perhaps more than other cultures, we seem to value how the look of rosy, plump cheeks convey a sense of robust health and a more youthful appearance.

Common name: cheek implants (malar augmentation)

What it does: Creates the illusion of higher cheek bones; adds greater definition to the cheek

Watch Out!
If an incision is made inside your mouth, your healing or recovery diet is likely to include only soft foods for the first few days—mashed potatoes, puddings, and simple warm soups. But be careful—a soft poppy-seed roll, chunky peanut butter, and small particles such as rice may become trapped, promoting bacteria and even infection! Rinsing your mouth with water after every meal will help.

Price range: $1,500 to $4,000
Operation duration: Less than an hour
Anesthetic: Local
The procedure:
Incisions are made inside the mouth above the upper gums and the surgeon positions the implant into place. Frequently, to anchor each implant, a piece of Gore-Tex, a fibrous material, is surgically glued to the back of the implant. Gore-Tex permits new fibroblasts to grow amid the intertwining material; the process somewhat knits the implant in place.

Understanding the aesthetics of the jaw

Skin that droops over the front part of the upper neck is usually what we call a double chin. This sagging is a result of a combination of sagging neck skin, the accumulation of fat, and the loss of muscle tone.

The operation done to tighten this sagging tissue is called a submental lipectomy, or a chin tuck, which is the removal of fat, eliminating the double chin. It is often preferable to leave some looseness in the skin of the neck to match the rest of the face and to prevent it from looking unnatural. However, for many prospects, a full neck lift may bring about the desired changes (see Chapter 9).

In chin enlargement or augmentation mentoplasty, a solid silicone implant is inserted on top of the chin bone, creating a more pronounced chin. The implant is inserted through an incision inside the lower lip or just under the chin. Excess fat and skin can also be removed during mentoplasty to help eliminate a sagging or double chin. Implants give a more natural result as they enhance the front and sides of the chin. The implant can be modified if you're unhappy with the overall appearance.

In another technique done to augment the chin, the lower part of the chin bone can be sawed off and moved forward. This is done through an incision that is made in the gum below the front teeth. This procedure, called a sliding genioplasty, can be done in place of a chin implant. The surgery is far more complex; the bone is secured with screws and the teeth are wired shut for weeks while the jaw bone heals. A sliding genioplasty, on the other hand, is a relatively simple procedure in which an incision is made in the mandible below the roots of the teeth, and the bony segment is advanced forward to augment the chin. The bony segment is wired to the stable portion of the jaw. Teeth are generally wired together when large segments of the mandible or maxilla are moved either forward or back. Keeping these variables in mind, here are the major chin corrections that are best served by a plastic or orthognathic surgeon.

Moneysaver
Chin augmentation is sometimes done at the same time as a nose job. But because a small chin can make the nose look larger than it actually is, some people decide to undergo chin augmentation first before deciding on a nose job. After the chin has healed, the nose may look smaller than it did before the chin enlargement.

Common name: weak chin enlargement (mentoplasty, which is inserting an implant; or sliding genioplasty, which is repositioning bone)

What it does: Augmentation gives greater prominence to the chin; repositioning enhances other features

Price range: $1,500 to $6,000

Operation duration: 30 minutes or slightly longer

Anesthetic: Local, or local with sedation (MAC) for bone work

The procedure:

Originally, augmenting a weak or receding chin involved grafts of living bone or cartilage, which had the unfortunate tendency to decrease in size as the body absorbed the newly placed material. Implants, now used nearly universally, have replaced grafts, and most are made of medical-grade silicone. Implants may be already sized to fit or carved to the desired shape by the surgeon.

Chin implants are typically placed through incisions in the skin just beneath the chin or inside the lower lip (see the following before and after photos). The lip incision leaves no external scars. Some surgeons, however, feel that the risk of infection around implants is higher, so they prefer to use the outside skin incision. The resulting scar is usually relatively inconspicuous. Like so many issues relating to cosmetic surgery, there's an opposing group of surgeons who disagree, preferring to use the lip incision. Consult with your surgeon to determine the best approach for you.

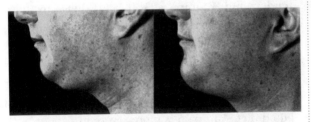

A chin implant, accompanied by modest liposuction, gives greater definition and harmony to the jaw line. (Source: Dr. Gregory LaTrenta)

Another chin implant—actually a combination of implants along each side of the jaw—adds bulk to a pointy or very sharp jawbone. An internal incision is made on either side of the lower lip and, again, pockets are fashioned to hold the implants in place, which give a more rugged, square-jaw appearance. Dressings are not usually necessary.

Watch Out!
Large chin implants tend to develop more postoperative complications than smaller ones. Ask to see the range of implants and be sure your doctor quantifies the relative size of your proposed implant.

Most cosmetic surgeons find that as many as 15 to 25 percent of cosmetic nose surgery prospects could benefit from chin augmentation. This percentage is somewhat lower for candidates for face lifts, which tend to restore the clean jaw line obscured by sagging skin.

Postoperative expectations:

Most implant patients experience mild discomfort; the equivalent to very minor dental work. Those who have had small implants placed through an outside incision generally have less discomfort, though a certain tightness might prevail for several days. If external sutures are used, these are often removed in three days or so; healing progresses very well for most patients. The external scar invariably fades within about three months. In most cases the scar is camouflaged in a natural skin fold.

Incisions in the mouth may be slightly more tender and require a soft-food diet—no hard chewing—to promote a speedy recovery. Shaving may be postponed in the area for several days. Protect your health and investment: Keep your fingers off the implant! Patients with wired jaws must follow their doctor's protocol fastidiously, including following a liquid diet. And pain is more severe in patients with wired jaws, though the pain usually subsides within a week and can be remedied with medication.

Possible complications:

In rare instances, infection may develop; fastidious oral hygiene must be strictly followed. Infection is most likely to occur if the jaw has been wired or the implant incision is inside the mouth. Injury can move the implant and some patients develop an abundance of scar tissue, though this is uncommon. Other implant complications include bleeding, displacement, infection, extrusion, unsatisfactory scarring, chronic pain, and dissatisfaction with results.

If your implant moves slightly during healing, it may *feel* somewhat crooked beneath the skin. However, in most instances, the appearance of the chin is perfectly fine; there is no need to reposition the implant. In some cases, artificial implants have gradually eroded the bone of the chin, causing recession to recur. This is less apt to happen if the implant is placed on top of the membrane that nourishes the bone, called the *periosteum*, rather than below this support tissue.

Unofficially...
If the implant must be removed, don't immediately despair. In some cases, newly formed scar tissue can create its own prominence, so the operation may not have to be repeated.

Common name: chin reduction (chin osteotomy)

What it does: Reduces the exaggerated chin thrust that often detracts from other facial features

Price range: $2,500 to $6,000

Operation duration: Several hours or less

Anesthetic: Usually general, but varies according to the correction required

The procedure:

Unlike chin augmentation, reducing prominence along the jaw line is far more surgically demanding. There are several options. If the teeth line up in a fairly normal manner—what dentists call the bite—the chin can be reduced in size by cutting down the prominent portion. Some surgeons prefer to excise a segment of bone from this area and slide the chin back, again using wires to close the jaw and to maintain position during healing.

When evaluating your chin, a good surgeon must scrutinize your entire profile. Dental models will also be prepared during the preoperative period. A secondary procedure may be necessary to complete facial harmony. In some cases, chin abnormality may significantly affect features. Another adjunct operation can substantially enhance your final appearance, so your surgeon may be quite justified in pointing this out—even if you were not previously aware of it.

The second method involves separating the chin bone from the tooth-bearing portion of the jaw, removing a portion of this bone, and placing the jaw in a more backward position. This requires that the reshaped area be held in place by wiring. An advantage is that the chin does not have to be sculpted. But, depending on the correction to be made, drains may be needed to remove excess fluids from the site.

Postoperative expectations:

After the operation, pulse, blood pressure, and breathing are carefully monitored until you can return to your hospital room. Discharge from the hospital is usually on the second postoperative day. Your head is continually elevated and cold compresses help to reduce swelling. Some surgeons prescribe cortisone-like medication to minimize swelling.

Postoperative pain can be significant, and medicine is given to ease it. Elastic bands or wires make it difficult, if not impossible, to speak.

Vomiting is a dangerous early risk; any nausea must be vigilantly observed. Since your mouth is wired, any vomiting that occurs may enter the lungs, bringing on pneumonia. Medicine is administered at the first sign of nausea, and, as an additional safeguard, wire cutters are kept on your night stand.

With your jaw wired shut, adequate nutrition must be delivered through an intravenous line.

Unofficially...
To give the chin the best improvement, another correction may include orthodontic treatment to normalize your bite. Remember: In no case can chin surgery substitute for problems with teeth position.

Within a day or so, and for at least six to eight weeks, you'll take food—only liquids, many high-calorie—through your mouth. But unbelievably, you'll learn to do this without opening it!

Before leaving the hospital, you'll learn how to use mouth antiseptics frequently and the proper methods of cleaning the teeth and gums.

Watch Out!
With jaw surgery, despite the intake of high-calorie liquids, you may drop a clothes size or more. There is frequently a 10- or 20-pound weight loss.

If small rubber drains were inserted into the incisions, these are removed on the first postoperative day. Skin stitches are usually removed on the third to fifth postoperative day, and the healing wound may be supported with skin tape for a while. When the wires are removed (six to eight weeks), the jaw will feel stiff; chewing solid foods should be slowly reintroduced. Sometimes warm compresses can help ease stiffness.

Possible complications:

In contrast to adding heft to the chin, this opposing procedure—reducing chin size—unfortunately has a somewhat higher rate of failure. The soft tissue (overlying the chin) may not sufficiently line up with the bone and the over-shot position may emerge. This is sometimes precipitated by developing scar tissue. However, a highly qualified orthognathic surgeon can give you a reasonable assessment of this likelihood during your consultation and tell you what secondary measures may be required.

Another complication is infection. If it cannot be readily controlled with antibiotics, early removal of the wires may be required. This may result in incomplete healing of the bone, causing abnormal mobility, and require an additional procedure to foster the bony union.

Bright Idea
Excessive swelling in the early postoperative period may interfere with breathing and thus require some breathing support. If you have sinus trouble or tend to suffer from nasal stuffiness, alert your surgeon beforehand; he can prescribe medicine that can help you breathe more easily.

Injury to the nerve that supplies the lower teeth and lips may produce lip numbness, usually temporary, but it can be permanent. Nerve damage is more common in procedures that are performed on the tooth-bearing portion of the jaw.

Lip and mouth considerations

The mouth area, notably the lips and the smile lines, can achieve improvement with simple procedures. For example, the facial creases or indents that run from the nostrils to the corners of the lips are called the *nasolabial folds*. These folds accommodate the movement of the face by folding inward when a person smiles. They are a natural part of every person's face. With age, the folds may become more pronounced, but many young people have significant creases as well. Plastic surgeons have developed several techniques to reduce the depth of these folds. Not all, however, can guarantee a completely even outcome. Most lip and nasolabial corrections involve augmentation; others rely on surgical corrections, such as the following lip procedure.

Common name: lip enhancement through reposition of upper and lower lip

What it does: Provides greater definition and plumps thin lips

Price range: $1,500 to $5,000

Operation duration: About 40 minutes per lip

Anesthetic: Local or local with sedation (MAC)

The procedure:

This is a relatively simple procedure, but one that demands great aesthetic talent and highly evolved surgical skill. An incision is made along the line where the rosy-colored part of the lip meets the skin—it's called the *vermilion border*. A tiny strip of white skin is removed and the red lip edge is advanced outward and stitched in place. For the most part, the incisions heal quickly and scars become imperceptible. The procedure usually provides the most satisfactory results to patients who have experienced thinning of the lips due to age.

Postoperative expectations:

In many cases, the mouth has a unique ability to heal quickly because of the ample blood supply to the area. The amount of pain may vary according to each patient's threshold. However, a surprising number of patients report no significant, enduring pain. Most discomforts—and the scratchiness of any protruding suture threads—are easily tolerated. Mild painkillers are often prescribed. The treated lip—which has probably been sutured with dissolving stitches—may show some bruising and swelling that can be treated with cold compresses or as directed by your surgeon. Usually a liquid or soft diet is prescribed to help the area heal quickly during the first few days.

Postoperative complications:

Typically there are few complications associated with this procedure. Some bleeding can occur and there are rare instances of mild infections. Both of these developments can usually be remedied almost immediately. However, for the best aesthetic result, the surgeon should be carefully selected and able to demonstrate solid expertise in this area.

Common name: lip implants

What it does: A soft, thread-like implant adds bulk to the top of the lip

Price range: $750 to $1,000 per area

Operation duration: Less than 20 minutes per implant

Anesthetic: Local with a nerve blocker

The procedure:

Two years or so ago, skinny Gore-Tex implants created great lip expectations. More threadlike in design, it, unfortunately, did not deliver good results. There was a tendency for implant threads to migrate within the lip; several women reported their implants popped out at the corner of the mouth while dining. One woman luckily had a small scissors with her; she trimmed the nuisance and proceeded to finish her crème brûlée. Other patients experienced another problem—as scar tissue formed and enveloped the thread, the pliant material could fold back on itself and create an unattractive bump or irregular shape.

Now, through an innovative new twist on this concept, far better results are now possible. The new material is manufactured by Collagen Corporation, and is more commonly known as the SoftForm Implant. It comes in two degrees of thickness—2.4 mm and 3.2 mm. The threads are tubular and have a notch in them. The notch accommodates fibroblasts that develop during healing; these twisting fibroblasts enter the notch opening and weave the implant in place from within. The scar tissue that develops outside also anchors the implant and the resulting added heft is natural looking.

The thread is surgically sealed in a cartridge delivery system, much like an ear piercing device, so there is no possibility of contamination. The surgeon makes two small incisions for the implant to enter and exit. Then the surgeon "injects" the implant. Being able to manipulate the implant from each opening helps give the best aesthetic result. Both incisions are closed with a small suture.

Unofficially...
Introduced in late 1998, the SoftForm Implant costs the surgeon about $275 apiece. After paying the manufacturer, doctors, in all fairness, pass along a healthy markup to each patient and charge from $500 to $750 for each implant. Since each lip requires at least two implants, add the surgery fee, and you can see why this fast augmentation can easily cost $2,000.

Postoperative expectations:

There is usually no bruising, and most patients find that they are back to normal within a week. The mouth feels much like dental work has been done, remaining numb for several hours; iced compresses can reduce swelling. Most prospects can talk and eat comfortably a few hours following the procedure. Because the implant material lasts indefinitely, the shape and fullness of your lips are enhanced permanently as the following before and after photos indicate.

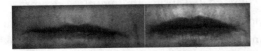

Before and after results indicate how the SoftForm Implant adds fullness. (Source: Dr. Sue Ellen Cox)

Many doctors who have pioneered the application feel the inventor's claim of a 75 percent improvement is somewhat exaggerated. Most see less, about 40 percent or so improvement.

Possible complications:

The procedure has produced few complications and remains too new to determine all risks. Infection is usually obviated by an oral antibiotic. Cold sore and herpes sufferers may require supplemental medication before undergoing this minor operation.

Common name: lip reduction

What it does: Reduces protruding lips

Price range: $1,500 to $4,500

Operation duration: Usually less than one and one-half hours

Anesthetic: Local with sedation (MAC)

The procedure:

Lip reduction to diminish an abnormally large, protuberant lower or upper lip is another procedure that has been criticized for removing ethnic qualities; although I have seen a wide cross section of ethnic patients who opt for this correction. Prospects should have a clear understanding of how much their mouth shape will be modified. Using a computer imaging system, a surgeon's sketch or rendering, or even obtaining a plaster cast of the face and filing the mouth area down can help you determine what looks best. Many reduction incisions can be accommodated inside the mouth and no scars are evident. A tiny strip of mucous membrane from the inner lip is removed and the edge is sutured in place. For the most part, the incisions heal quickly and dissolving sutures are often used.

If you are planning this surgery, be especially cautious when choosing your surgeon. Choose a surgeon who is experienced in performing the procedure, and seek every clarification that the result is something you will be happy with.

Postoperative expectations:

Depending on how much skin has been excised and your individual pain threshold, varying degrees of throbbing discomfort can be expected. Cold compresses and shaved iced chips reduce swelling and deliver a certain numbness. The sutures within the mouth can be bothersome, especially during the early stages of swelling.

Possible complications:

Like any operation that involves cutting away flesh, too much can be removed, resulting in unevenness, unwanted scar tissue inside the mouth, and possible nerve damage.

Timesaver
The mouth and lip areas have a remarkable ability to heal quickly. You can streamline the process with fastidious oral hygiene for the entire healing period. Use simple ice compresses for the first 24 hours—20 minutes on the swelling, 20 minutes off—as often as possible during that time.

Common name: reducing laugh lines (nasolabial fold)

What it does: Reduces the skin indent or crevice that typically runs from the base of the nose toward the outer corner of the mouth

Price range: $1,000 to $3,000

Operation duration: About one hour

Anesthetic: Local

The procedure:

The SoftForm Implant is also being used to plump up the nasal lines around the mouth. However, deep wrinkles and creases will not respond well to these new implants. Another technique uses muscle and tissue from another part of the body; the surgeon threads this into the folds by way of incisions made at the corners of the mouth and at the top of the folds near the nostril or just inside the nostril. A blood supply may grow into the transplanted tissue and result in a permanent change. Some doctors will partially liquefy the tissue and inject it with a large-sized needle. This may not last because a blood supply may not be established in the tissue.

Another technique uses surgical threads made out of a natural glycerin protein. This suture material is the same that is used to sew up interior organs during major surgery. Within several months the threads dissolve into the body. Some doctors say that the body replaces them with its own healing natural collagen that plumps the crevice. If the fold on each side of your mouth is significant, a modified face lift may be the best remedy (see Chapter 7).

The doctor may also use collagen to fill in nasolabial folds by injecting it into the skin; this is covered in the following section.

Postoperative expectations:

Most patients mention few, if any, uncomfortable reactions. There is some bruising and a mild amount of swelling. These tend to vanish within two days or so. The incision is virtually imperceptible; the small suture is not obvious to the eye and is removed within several days, depending on what your surgeon feels is best for your correction. Most patients resume normal activities the following day and are pleased with the results.

Postoperative complications:

There have been few postoperative complications reported. This may be in part because the procedure is relatively new. Some patients are somewhat disappointed that the resulting correction is not as significant as they had hoped for.

Together with your doctor, choose which lines to smooth and explain the type of results you would like. Be sure to have this discussion during your consultation and allergy test.

One of the leading manufacturers, Collagen Corporation, introduced this procedure nearly two decades ago. They call the injections implants, perhaps to offset the procedure's image of being only temporary. Collagen fades and is reabsorbed by the body within months; the manufacturer offers several formulations. You should know how each performs:

- Zyderm 1 and Zyderm 2 are used to treat fine lines, shallow scars, and thin-skinned areas.

- Zyplast is used to treat pronounced scars, lines, and furrows, as well as to define the lip border.

Zyplast is a form of injectable collagen that is cross-linked with the chemical glutaraldehyde to strengthen the collagen fibers. It is administered by

Unofficially...
The amount of collagen required to smooth a line varies from person to person and depends on many factors, including skin condition, general circulation, and amount of sun damage.

an injection with a fine gauge needle just beneath the surface of the skin.

Zyderm and Zyplast remain the leading injectable collagen products in the world and have been more rigorously tested than most other injectables. Because collagen is partly water, the injections are slightly overdone to make up for the water loss that will take place. There may be some swelling in the area where the collagen was injected, but this usually subsides within a few days. Healing takes anywhere from three to ten days. For a few days, men should avoid shaving the area where the injection took place.

Another collagen process involves cultivating cells from a patient's own dermis to grow additional collagen. A small punch biopsy of skin is obtained from behind the patient's ear and is sent to a laboratory where the collagen producing cells are cultivated.

Three cautions about injections:

First: In some collagen manufacturing, human cadavers are used for production. Cadaveric tissue is purchased from tissue banks and, once processed, this material can then be injected into lines and wrinkles to replace the body's own natural collagen. The procedures for donor screening (and serologic and microbiologic testing) of human cadaver collagen follow the federally mandated tissue recovery guidelines and those of the American Association of Tissue Banks. However, regulations do not require clinical studies to prove either the safety or the efficacy of the product. In my opinion, it's wise to stay with the leading manufacturers who do rigorous testing and clinical studies.

Be certain your doctor can provide literature from the manufacturer that fully details how the

Watch Out!
To maintain the results, repeat collagen injections are required. One caution: The more injections, the greater the potential for unwanted scar tissue. Injections of collagen should avoid the paper-thin skin around the eyes, where any lumps or scars that may develop will be obvious.

injectable material he or she recommends has been processed. Do not proceed with injections until you have read about the potential risks.

Second: Beware of injectable liquid silicone! There are questionable sources—some aesthetic spas or beauty clinics—that readily dispense silicone rather than pay the manufacturers' full rate for the rigorously tested collagen. Occasionally, an underground report surfaces about a new alternative clinic or facility that uses silicone for injections, claiming the results are long-lasting.

Here are five dangerous potential risks of silicone that these spas never inform you about:

1. Liquid silicone can easily travel throughout the body's system.

2. Should it settle in any of the organs, silicone can create havoc.

3. Silicone can contribute to ailments such as arthritis, immune disorders, rashes, hardening of the tissues, and breathing problems.

4. Silicone can wrap around nerves and marbleize within the skin and surrounding tissues, causing loss of sensation.

5. There can be hideous long-term complications, including tumors.

Third: When a patient's own fat is used, the process is called *fat transfer injections* or *autologous fat transplant.* The process is practically identical to collagen injections. However, there are no long-term studies that prove the procedure is safe and efficacious. For this reason, fat injections—often used to plump the back of aging hands or to fill out facial creases—remain controversial.

Bright Idea
Keep a written record of the name of the company that produced your injected collagen, the inventory batch control number, and the date of your procedure. Do this for each session. This information will be part of your permanent records—ask for a copy.

Common name: collagen and fat injections

What it does: Smoothes skin imperfections such as minor indented scars, wrinkles, folds, and shallow creases

Price range: $75 to $100 for test dose, $300 to $2,000 per session thereafter

Operation duration: Typically less than half an hour for smaller areas; up to one hour for larger areas; up to one hour or more for fat injections because additional time is needed to harvest the fat

Anesthetic: Local or local with sedation (MAC)

The procedure:

Four weeks prior to a collagen procedure, doctors administer a simple skin sensitivity test to determine if a patient has a sensitivity to the injectable collagen. The full injection procedure itself usually includes lidocaine to diminish discomfort. Ninety-seven percent of men and women tested have no allergic reaction to either collagen or lidocaine.

Because the patient's own fat is used, there is no chance that the patient will have a reaction to a fat injection. The fat is liposuctioned from the belly or thighs, then placed in tubes and mechanically spun to clarify it and separate the blood. The clarified fat is then injected into the part of the body that is to be filled out or enlarged. A syringe with a large-sized needle is used so the fat sustains as little damage as possible. A stitch or two may be required to close the donor site.

Postoperative expectations:

Recovery varies from patient to patient. If the area you have treated is small, the overcorrection will be less noticeable and you can return to work with little swelling or discomfort. More extensive treatments require a longer time to recover. The same is true for fat injections. In most cases, there will be some bruising that will fade, along with residual swelling.

Possible complications:

For the most part, under the supervision of a surgeon or dermatologist, collagen injections—as well as fat injections—are safe. I have seen some blistering on the lip area, and overcorrection can create an unnatural but temporary lumpiness. The fat process may be done by a cosmetic surgeon or dermatologist, but understand that many plastic surgeons deplore fat injections. They claim results are more fleeting than collagen. The blood that nourished the fat is removed in the transfer and without this vascular synergy, the body absorbs the fat cells or they die off. The desired result is lost within weeks or months. In rare cases, the fat may also create an odd appearance by reabsorbing unevenly or leaving bumps that do not smooth out. Subsequent surgery may not revise these imperfections. However, a number of other well-established doctors refute the temporary results and have presented a long list of satisfied patients who do indeed swear by the fat transfer benefits. Discuss options with your doctor to find out what procedure is best for you.

Just the facts

- You have only one face; if you seek to modify any features, choose small, incremental changes.

- Always weigh the risks of recovery and how you'll look; a face can't be hidden under clothing.

- Choose only a qualified surgeon who specializes in the procedure you seek.

- Get a clear idea of how long it will be before your face begins to look normal; plan accordingly.
- If you elect to have injections to smooth out imperfections, make certain your surgeon uses supplies from a tested, national manufacturer.

Upper/Lower Body and Skin Corrections

GET THE SCOOP ON...
How safe are breast implants? ▪ A rundown of
the most innovative breast and pectoral
implant procedures ▪ Procedures that lift or
reduce heavy breasts ▪ Shaping the upper arms
with underarm liposuction ▪ Tummy tucks for a
slimmer profile

PART V

Procedures for the Chest, Abdomen, and Arms

F or several practical purposes, breasts might be better off on one's back. Breast feeding, for example, could be done while the busy mother uses her free hands for other tasks. Of course, the all-important early infant bonding might never be adequately developed. (And the critically important breast self-exam would hardly be routine.) If, at times, the human body is an impractical contraption, it nevertheless remains one of the more effective ways to communicate who we are. For example, in the late 19th century, a prosperous man often deliberately gained weight to underscore his wealth. A potbelly was the perfect way to show off an expensive gold chain that traversed from end to end, attaching itself to an expensive gold pocket watch.

Today, for both sexes, the physical attributes of the upper body remain a meaningful currency: a

255

lean, upright posture, accented by a reasonably developed, upright bosom (for women) or buffed pectoral area (for men), can signal many things— attractiveness, health, even self-esteem. If these attributes were insignificant, the procedures you'll read about in this chapter would never have been developed.

Breast implants

While many people know that silicone implants were banned, they are confused by what type of implant is currently offered. And, they wonder, is it safe? If it's a saline implant, why does it also have silicone? Today's approved implants are made of silicone rubber envelopes; these sacs are filled with a saline solution. Saline-filled implants are *not* the same as the silicone gel implants that were used previously but are now prohibited for cosmetic-only purposes by the Food and Drug Administration.

Those banned silicone implants created a major controversy 10 years ago when women began complaining of varied symptoms, ranging from mild nausea and achy joints to severe suffering that included heavy scar formation around the implants, arthritis, and serious flu-like symptoms. Leaking implants ravaged the body and the talk-show circuit was rife with women claiming hideous, life-threatening results. The qualitative findings seemed to suggest the implants represented serious risk, and they were withdrawn from the market.

Many surgeons look back on the previous implants' sturdiness and performance with nostalgia; those implants, in their collective opinion, were predictably reliable and worked like a charm. To them, silicone implants are safe and remain the gold standard. This opinion is clearly not shared by many of the women who have or have had problems with silicone breast implants. A number of leading medical journals explored the efficacy and safety of silicone implants and could not identify the equivalent of the harmful findings being claimed by many women in the marketplace. In sum, the findings echo what silicone implant supporters always maintained; there was no medical correlation that could be tied to the symptoms claimed by women who had implants.

Before considering implants, there are two warnings to all prospects:

1. Never, ever entertain augmenting your breasts if there is any evidence of family breast cancer.

2. Implants may prevent one of the most important tests designed to protect you—the mammography—from delivering clear, readable results.

If you consult with a surgeon about having implants, be sure to thoroughly discuss the doctor's history of performing implants and ask how many of his patients have had problems. Any initial consultation should also cover a thorough discussion of all the issues, with straight answers to the following questions:

■ What is currently known about an association of autoimmune disease with breast or pectoral implants?

■ What is the possibility of rupture, what are the signs to watch for, and what is involved if your implants rupture?

■ What is the surgeon's understanding of capsular contracture (the tightening of scar tissue that forms around implants) and how might it affect you?

- Might additional corrective surgeries be needed?

- How is mammography testing (and interpretation of results) likely to be compromised?

Watch Out!
Although significant complications are quite rare, there is no way to predict if you will have two or more of the serious reactions.

In varying degrees, capsule formation—sometimes also called capsular contracture—invariably occurs in all breast augmentations. There are three stages that may occur and each requires your attention. They are: (1) the breast looks normal but feels unnaturally firm; (2) the breast looks abnormal—the capsule has contracted, distorting the implant into a hard ball; and (3) the breast looks abnormal, the capsule has contracted, and it is painful.

Usually, if you develop the first capsule condition, no treatment is recommended. For the second type—abnormal appearance—the usual protocol calls for the incision to be reopened and the capsule released. There is a chance that this contraction may recur. The third problem, contraction plus pain, usually requires repositioning the implant. If pain persists, have the implants removed.

Here are the basic operation approaches for breast augmentation.

Common name: breast implants (augmentation mammoplasty)

What it does: Increases breast size and may reshape contour

Price range: $2,500 to $8,000

Operation duration: Usually less than one and a half hours

Anesthetic: Local with sedation (MAC)

The procedure:

Today, this procedure requires very small incisions, in relation to the size of most implants. Incisions are most frequently made in three common areas:

around the lower half of the areola; under the breasts (in the natural inframammary fold); or in the armpit. Some surgeons use an endoscope for inserting implants through a small incision in the armpit, making the entry site increasingly popular. It had recently fallen out of favor because implants appeared too high and unnatural. Previously, implants placed through the armpit were maneuvered into position by a blunt instrument that looked like a miniature hockey stick. Getting the implant in place required a great deal of pushing, and most surgeons were not pleased with the final results. The endoscope lets the surgeon see exactly where the implant rests, delivers far better results, and generates less bruising and swelling.

Another innovative technique developed by plastic surgeon Gregory La Trenta, MD, injects the breast sac with a liquid that causes tumescent swelling. Once the skin is stretched in this manner, the implant can be inserted with less trauma. Bruising and bleeding are minimized and the patient endures less pain throughout recovery. Normal skin tone returns almost immediately.

Today, the implant is positioned behind existing breast tissue, either in front of or behind the pectoral muscles. The implant is centered beneath the nipple. Placing the implant under the breast muscle permits a clear mammography reading.

Once the implants are correctly positioned, the surgeon delicately sutures the incisions. Some stitches dissolve; others are removed a few days after surgery. Protective surgical tape may be applied to the incisions. You will experience swelling; some patients upon awakening immediately think that the implants are too big. As swelling is reduced, you will feel more comfortable with your new shape.

Watch Out!
The increased breast mound and depth of cleavage are determined by the size of the implant. Be sure to see and approve each implant size prior to surgery.

The following photos show how augmentation can enhance a bosom.

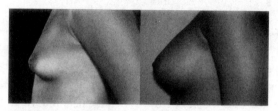

Before and after implant results; the incisions were made under the arms. (Source: Dr. Z. Paul Lorenc)

There should be little disruption of the mammary ducts; you should be able to breast-feed. Some temporary loss of the sensory nerves is common and is a result of the area having been stretched to make room for the implant; sensation usually returns within three months.

Expect to wear a surgical bra, night and day (except when you shower) over the one- or two-week period after the procedure. Some women continue to tape incisions for an additional month to minimize scar widening. Expect some obvious restriction of upper body activity during this period.

Postoperative expectations:

Fluid or blood accumulation under the skin may resolve itself spontaneously or require surgical drainage. Excessive bleeding following the operation may cause swelling and pain. If this condition occurs, a second operation may be required to control the bleeding, but this is quite rare. Keep all medications and comfort items within easy reach, on a night stand or close by.

Stitches, depending on type and location, are removed in a week or so. The patient should sleep in an upright position, propped comfortably with soft pillows. For the first few months some women experience greater swelling and breast discomfort during their menstrual cycles. Scars will be firm and pink for six to eight weeks, and fade to pale after a year.

Possible complications:

Complications are rare but may include rupture of the implant, often traceable to an injury. If a saline-filled implant breaks, the bag will deflate within a few hours and the salt water will be absorbed by the body. Immediately alert your surgeon; replacement is a straightforward procedure. In some cases, infection does flare up. This can be controlled through prescriptions, but *always* dictates removal of the implant. Adhesions near the scars can create lumpiness, itching, and discomfort. If the bumps become significant, your surgeon may control them with a cortisone injection or they may have to be surgically corrected.

Common name: chest buffing or pectoral implants

What it does: Adds bulk to the male chest, often creating greater definition

Price range: $3,000 to $6,000

Operation duration: Usually less than one and a half hours

Anesthetic: Usually local

The procedure:

Inserted through an auxiliary incision—in the armpit—chest implants are positioned above the male nipple to fill out the upper chest. They provide definition to the upper pectoralis muscles or may be used to camouflage bulging grooves resulting from a tear in this muscle.

Care should be taken to select an appropriate-size pectoral implant; excessively large implants make the torso appear stumpy rather than sleek.

Unofficially...
Female competitive body builders who seek enhanced cleavage often opt for pectoral implants rather than traditional breast implants, which appear too round and bulbous for their lean, fibrous chests. The slope of male pectoral implants imparts a more natural look.

Men's physical reactions to pectoral implants are the same as those experienced by women who have had breast implants. Men should discuss potential reactions, as outlined previously, with their surgeon prior to surgery.

Postoperative expectations:

Bright Idea
Select a plastic surgeon who is widely experienced in pectoral implants. And most important: Be sure to speak with former patients and get their reactions to the results.

Men can expect a certain amount of bruising, which tends to be minor and dissipates a few days after surgery. Swelling creates a good deal of discomfort and is managed by applying cold compresses. The area can ache considerably on the first day (and for the first week). Many patients liken the discomfort to that of an intense, high-level workout. Others claim greater pain and are uncomfortable not being able to turn their upper torso during the first few days. Soft clothing should be worn. Upper body stiffness will pass within a week or 10 days. Absolutely no physical activity should be undertaken until your surgeon tells you it is safe to do so.

Possible complications:

Some qualitative information seems to suggest that men have a higher level of implant complications. Most of these cases seem to stem from lax recovery follow-through. I know of six individual serious pectoral implant infection cases; unbelievably, all involved patients swimming, sunbathing, and even playing volleyball on sandy beaches before recovery was complete.

The procedure can deliver uneven results or a disappointing or modest amount of augmentation. The major complications, apart from infection, are collections of fluid, even blood, around the implant; displacement of the implants; or even a pointy corner of the implant that protrudes from under the skin.

If patients follow their doctor's instructions and allow plenty of time for recovery, most pectoral implants have no complications and bear good results.

Breast lift and reduction approaches

There are a number of reasons why breasts sag—the natural process of aging, the result of breast-feeding, weight fluctuations, or having exceptionally large breasts to begin with. Many women accept sagging as a natural response, while for others, the physical nuisance can be quite significant. Rashes, skin tags, and other dermatological flare-ups can plague the area. For others, a flaccid, drooping breast brings on a psychological despair that erodes self-esteem. The most common reason why a woman's chest loses its bounce and firmness has much to do with how the breast is constructed. A woman's breasts are made of:

- Fatty deposits
- Tissue
- Underlying support muscles

The muscle that holds the bosom in place has many demands placed on it. Significant weight gain, exceptional physical activity and bouncing, medications, and nursing all tax the underlying support system. Additionally, as we age, the body loses muscle mass each year.

For these reasons, the following two operations can provide women with greater comfort and satisfaction.

Common name: breast reduction (reduction mammoplasty)

What it does: Reduces the size of a heavy, cumbersome bosom and, in older women, can restore the natural lift of the bosom

Price range: $5,500 to $10,000

Operation duration: Three to four hours

Anesthetic: General

The procedure:

In breast reduction, your plastic surgeon reduces the size of your breasts, but aesthetic expertise is required to sculpt and shape them. Candidates can be very young or mature adults, even seniors. Breast reduction is almost always done under general anesthetic in a hospital. If large amounts of breast resection and associated blood loss are anticipated, you may be asked to donate a unit of your own blood one or two weeks prior to the operation.

The standard incision follows the keyhole pattern, which is:

1. A circle placed above the areola and nipple area

2. Vertical lines that fall from each side of this circle, creating an inverted "v" to the crease under the bosom

Fat and extra tissue are then removed; most extra tissue comes from the side and lower half of each breast. The dissection extends down to the muscles of the chest wall. This surgical depth explains why muscles feel so tender and sore after reduction surgery. The nipple, though still attached, is moved upward to the circle created by the incision and then sutured; the two sides that formed the inverted "v" are sutured together, making a firm, beautifully shaped smaller bosom. All other approaches are variations of this technique.

In extreme cases of breast reduction, a complete nipple graft may be necessary if the distance to the new nipple position is great. However, surgeons use this technique only when absolutely necessary, since sensation in the area is almost completely lost.

Both the nipple and areola are transferred as a skin graft to their new position and the graft permits regeneration of sensation; although this often takes several months at the very least.

A drain is placed on each side to carry old blood and fluid accumulation. These are usually left in place overnight or for a few days if drainage is excessive.

The incisions are sutured and taped. You will be placed in a surgical bra padded with gauze. Some women go home the same day, but others require a one-night hospital stay.

Postoperative expectations:

The pain is typically significant for the first two to three days, especially when you move or cough. You may be given breathing exercises to keep your lungs clear. You'll likely take narcotic pain medication for up to one week, when nondissolving sutures are removed. You will be sore for a week or longer, at which point any residual discomfort is easily controlled with over-the-counter medications.

No showers or baths are allowed; fresh tape is applied over the sutures. A sponge bath is permitted until the drains are removed. You will continue to wear the support bra night and day except when showering for the first two to three weeks. Sleeping, propped upright by pillows, may be slightly uncomfortable until your body adjusts.

Each woman's reaction is remarkably different, but all should plan a stress-free, easy schedule until normal strength and endurance have returned. It is wise to allow an absolute minimum of two *full* weeks before returning to work, which should be resumed slowly. When you return to work, avoid tight and uncomfortable upper garments, especially if you're

> O'er her warm cheek and rising bosom move The bloom of young Desire and purple light of Love.
> —Thomas Gray (1715–1771), *The Progress of Poesy*

exposed to warm temperatures. It is also recommended that you tape incisions for an additional month to minimize scar widening. Physical activity is restricted until your doctor approves it; absolutely no bouncing or upper body workouts for at least four weeks. The body must adequately heal itself inside. If your work is sedentary, you may be able to return after just one week.

Your surgeon may recommend that you take an iron supplement before surgery and for three months afterward to build up the iron in your body. Drink plenty of water and follow a healthy nutritional regimen. Try to avoid even a small weight loss or gain.

Possible complications:

Severe problems are rare, but do monitor your body's response carefully. Despite the significant pain, few women regret the procedure which can instantly relieve lower back pain, extreme pressure on both shoulders, and angry skin rashes. Your surgeon should alert you to any exceptional risks for your case. Fluid or blood accumulation under the skin may resolve itself spontaneously or require surgical drainage.

In some cases, scars should be taped for the first six weeks after surgery to prevent widening. Though permanent, they will fade over time. Scars are generally positioned so that they can be hidden easily by clothing. Pigmentation changes may become permanent if scars are exposed to the sun too soon after the operation. Loss of skin or even part (or all) of the nipple is greater for patients who smoke, as discussed in earlier chapters.

Common name: breast lift (mastopexy)

What it does: Repositions drooping breasts

Price range: $4,500 to $10,000

Moneysaver
Scars may widen or thicken, requiring revision at a later time. However, since this is usually due to tension placed on the incision, inexpensive, soft surgical tape can help reduce this stress. Wear this tape regularly whenever you move about.

Operation duration: Usually under two hours

Anesthetic: Local injection for small corrections; intravenous anesthetic for some cases; others may require general anesthetic

The procedure:

A breast lift won't keep your breasts firm forever. Gravity, pregnancy, aging, and weight fluctuations will eventually take their toll again. Better results have been reported by women who have implants along with their breast lift if they want to replace lost breast mass as well as lift their breasts.

There are several variations of incision placement. The most common uses the keyhole pattern described in the reduction procedure. This allows for reduction of the diameter of the areola as well as elevation of the nipple. Using this technique, the nipple can be raised several inches so that it is at the level of the rounded side crease, called the *inframammary fold,* or very slightly lower. This is a key aesthetic goal of a successful breast lift; otherwise, the nipple will point upward after healing.

No breast tissue is removed in mastopexy, only skin. Because of this, you will remain relatively the same size, although your breasts will be firmer and seem larger because your skin "bra" has been tightened.

In this operation, there is little disruption of the sensory nerves or the mammary ducts, so there is little risk of permanently affecting nipple sensation or the ability to subsequently breast-feed. You may be surprised that most women experience only moderate soreness rather than pain after this operation.

The following photos show before and after results and illustrate the aesthetic goal of raising the nipple so that it is in line with the inframammary fold.

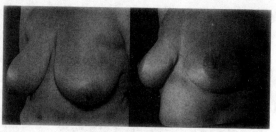

The discomfort of pendulous breasts is replaced by a lifted bosom which better matches this woman's proportions. (Source: Dr. Gregory LaTrenta)

Postoperative expectations:

Breasts will be bruised, swollen, and achy for two to three days following the operation. You will wear an elastic bandage or surgical bra over gauze dressings for three or four days. This will be replaced by a soft support bra that must be worn day and night for up to four weeks, though many women continue long after that. Nondissolving sutures will be removed after a week. Incisions are often taped (in some cases, up to six weeks) to reduce possible widening of scars.

Breast skin may be very dry following surgery and should be moisturized several times a day. Do not tug at your skin and do not apply this lotion to the sutured areas until all tape strips have separated.

Postoperative swelling may cause some loss of feeling in the nipples and numbness in the breast tissues. This will likely subside over the next six to eight weeks or longer.

Remember: As most women age, the ratio of fat to breast tissue increases. This has little to do with *being* fat, but rather is a reflection of the natural aging process. The more fat content in your breasts, the more your breasts will sag and the less firm they will be.

Possible complications:

Most patients endure little pain and recover quickly. If a hematoma develops, it can be treated by draining, though many resolve on their own. The most serious complication relates to the aesthetics of scarring and its inherent irregular pigmentation. A few women report a loss of sensation around the nipple; most feeling eventually does return.

Procedures for more beautiful arms and hands

Recently, underarm sculpting has made a significant leap in delivering satisfactory results. Fat in the upper arms can be a trait for many women. As women age, the underlying muscles become flaccid and can shake with the barest movement. Many young women, too, have this trait and find the aesthetics undesirable. When exercise does not correct the situation, two procedures—liposuction and skin excisions—can modify the fat and flaccid tissue. Recently, these two procedures have been combined with Endermologie, an innovative nonsurgical method from France. (Endermologie is covered in depth in Chapter 13.) This combination of procedures has delivered fine results for a variety of patients.

Common name: upper arm shaping (brachialectomy)

What it does: Removes flabby underarm skin, giving the arm a better shape

Price range: $2,000 to $3,500

Operation duration: Usually under two hours

Anesthetic: Local

The procedure:

An incision is made under the arm, near the armpit, and the upper area may be injected with a tumescent solution. The area is then liposuctioned. If excess skin must be excised, an incision of several inches is placed down the arm from armpit to elbow to remove what are sometimes called "batwings." This surgery leaves a scar, which will become less noticeable over time. The tightened area is then sutured closed.

If the person requires greater definition, Endermologie treatments (see Chapter 13) can be scheduled over a period of weeks or months until the arm has become more sculpted.

Postoperative expectations:

Tenderness in the armpit can make movement somewhat difficult for the first few days. There is usually minor bruising that subsides within the week. Some patients report achy shoulders that may be due to the area being manipulated. The arm area is bandaged to keep swelling down and help the skin contract. Sutures are removed in five or so days and the bandage is worn for several more weeks.

Possible complications:

There is the risk of infection, which can be managed with medication. If too much tissue has been removed, the area can appear somewhat hollow and deformed; discuss corrective measures with your surgeon.

Improving the appearance of hands

Because we are constantly moving and flexing our hands, they are not good candidates for cosmetic surgery. However, skin appearance can be made smoother and scars or brown spots removed or minimized through chemical peeling (see Chapter 6). Additionally, though fat transfer remains controversial—there are no long-term studies about its efficacy and safety—a number of surgeons support its use for plumping aging hands and diminishing the signs of protruding veins and bones. Costs for these treatments vary from several hundred to several thousands of dollars. With fat transfers, a series of treatments may be required to achieve and then maintain results.

Where flat is desirable

A slim profile is best delivered by a flat tummy. While age can mean a widening girth, many young people, too, seek an aesthetic improvement when a significant weight loss leaves them with a flabby tummy. In many cases, a series of exercises over the long term can produce wonderful results. Indeed, if the person is under 35, excess skin can eventually diminish, following a major weight loss. However, after a certain age, obesity takes its toll; if this person loses weight, the skin tone vanishes along with the excessive pounds. Depending on the amount of skin to be excised, two treatments can address a formerly heavy person's tummy concern. Many women opt for this correction following pregnancy.

Common name: tummy tuck (abdominoplasty)

What it does: Removes the excess wrinkled skin and fatty tissue from the abdomen and tightens abdominal muscles. The overall effect produces a smoother, flatter tummy.

Price range: $4,000 to $9,000

Operation duration: Depending on scope, less than two and a half hours. Smaller procedures can be accommodated in under one hour.

Anesthetic: General

The procedure:

Tummy tucks can be painful because the torso moves with every breath. It is major surgery and

Watch Out!
A tummy tuck should not be performed on candidates who remain seriously overweight. Due to the varied risks inherent to their lifestyle and weight, obese patients make poor candidates.

should always be done in a hospital, and may include an overnight hospital stay. The best candidate for this surgery has relatively normal weight, weak muscles, and excess skin. Patients who are considerably overweight may be advised to lose weight prior to surgery. When discussing potential results with your surgeon, bear in mind that your age and skin tone have a lot to do with the level of improvement you can expect.

This operation is performed through a crescent-like incision that is placed at the bottom of the tummy between the hip bones. An incision is also made around the belly button and the skin is lifted up (toward the rib cage) and away from the abdomen. The underlying muscles in the abdomen—in some patients, these muscles have separated—are tightened by sutures. Fatty deposits are removed and excess skin cut away. Because the skin is pulled downward, a new belly button opening has to be cut and the belly button repositioned. The incision is then closed and the skin is sewn around the belly button. Drainage tubes may be inserted and left in place for a day or more. Firm elastic dressings are applied.

Endoscopic tummy tucks:

In cases where the patient has only mild sagging, a less invasive operation may be possible using endoscopy, in which a small opening is made in the navel. The endoscopic approach is used in patients who require only tightening of muscles. This is not a recommended application for patients who have excess skin.

Like the traditional abdomnioplasty, another minituck is frequently combined with liposuction—which can be standard liposuction, tumescent, or UAL. (Liposuction is discussed in detail in Chapter 6.)

This procedure is further explained in the next chapter where liposuction plays a significant role in shaping the lower body.

Unlike the traditional abdominoplasty, the belly button is not repositioned, but an incision may be necessary to gather hanging skin. This procedure can address minor "bikini bulges" and is often sought by women following pregnancy. Despite a rigorous exercise program, their small "balloon" or "kangaroo pouch" is eradicated only by surgery. This procedure requires a shorter transverse incision, extending from one side of the groin to the other.

With both procedures, be warned that there are significant scar considerations. With standard abdominoplasty, you will have a single major scar across your lower abdomen, extending from hip to hip. You will also have a small scar around your belly button, which is moved to accommodate the lift. Still, the results can produce a lean, flat stomach, as you can see in the following before and after photos.

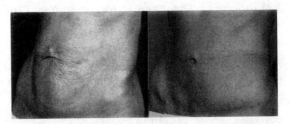

Toning the lower abdomen via a tummy tuck can be seen in this side-by-side comparison. Note that the patient's final scar is barely perceptible. (Source: Dr. Gregory LaTrenta)

With a miniabdominoplasty, if excision is required, a single scar will run across the pubic hairline.

Remember: Scars, though permanent, usually fade over time. You can expect it to take from nine months to a year for a scar to mature or start to pale. A longer time might be required for some patients. A skillful surgeon will make incisions where they are easily hidden under clothes and most bathing suits.

Postoperative expectations:

With either the traditional tummy tuck or the endoscopic tummy tuck, the surgery is major. Expect to feel sore and constricted; you'll want and need pain medication. The usual recovery time is from three to six weeks. Frequently, surgical drains are used for the first day or so after abdominoplasty and sometimes after lower-body reduction procedures (see Chapter 13).

You will also be significantly limited in what you can do during the first week. Guided by your physician, you can expect a progressive return to normal activity during the second through sixth weeks. But it can be months before you feel completely back to normal.

It takes time for the new shape to settle in, though results are obvious almost immediately. You'll be ready for a new wardrobe in about three months.

Possible complications:

As with all surgeries, there can be problems with healing, infection, and hemorrhaging. If too much fat is removed, the skin may not heal properly and parts of the skin may die (necrosis).

Just the facts

- Never seek breast implants if there is a trace of breast cancer in your family.

- Breast implants placed below the muscle provide clearer interpretation of future mammography results.

> "
> There's a great benefit from medical massage therapy, sometimes called *lymphatic drainage massage therapy* for many lower-body surgeries, beginning the second or third week after the operation. This therapy can dramatically relieve stiffness, circulation, and reduce swelling.
> —Timothy Callaghan, trained physical therapist, owner of Liberty Fitness
> "

- Upper-body surgery generally requires a carefully managed recovery period; don't plan to bounce right back to work.

- Tummy tucks can provide dramatic results, but neither the incision nor the surgery is minor.

- All upper-body surgery—arm liposuction, breast augmentation/reduction and abdominoplasty— yield the best results when normal weight is maintained.

The Lower Body: How to Get the Results You Want

I f we could all draw the contour we wanted for our bodies, many would want to resketch the lower contours. Unlike many cultures, notably European ones, Americans have always been fairly limited about how much fat they feel is appropriate to carry on the lower extremities. It may be our athletic high standards or the ever-looming California surfer ideal that dictate these guidelines. But, for the most part, we also equate a hefty bottom with sloth and a lack of determination. In order to modify her thick calves and thick ankles, millionairess Betty Hutton endured some of the most painfully crippling surgery possible. Done more than five decades ago, the results were negligible.

Today, the lower body can be more effectively reshaped. (Although the calves, for the most part, being more fibrous rather than just fatty, can benefit only so much from liposuction.)

In this chapter, you'll learn why liposuction for the lower body is somewhat different—the areas are bigger and more prone to postoperative lumpiness, even when care is taken. Also, after liposuction, an infection can race through the new tunnel where fat has been removed, delivering dangerous results. Still, when carefully managed, the majority of patients are enormously satisfied and emerge healthy and happy. Many would easily repeat the process and pay more to maintain their new comely contour where previously difficult, bulging pockets were evident. Three varied approaches, with a fourth emerging technique called Endermologie, are effectively being refined to treat buttocks, thighs, knees, and calves. Here's what you need to know.

Some basics about liposuction and your lower body

There are several good news bulletins about down under. Liposuction is making quantum leaps in delivering superior results with less trauma—bruising, swelling, and loss of blood—to the treated area. After surgery and recovery, bottoms and legs are more streamlined, smooth, and less likely to show the imperfect lumping that accompanied earlier operations. And, for the most part, skilled surgeons can hide many of the required incisions in natural body folds.

Not surprising, with all the improvements and changes, controversy emerges. Which technique is best for the lower body? A newly emerging, non-surgical approach called Endermologie is getting positive press, and some surgeons use it in tandem with liposuction.

Could this approach replace surgery? Some say yes, others say no. To understand the benefits of

Unofficially...
Endermologie was developed in France where early liposuction operations were refined several decades ago.

Endermologie, you first must understand current liposuction basics. After fully examining what liposuction can and cannot do, you can better appreciate how Endermologie can serve as an adjunct procedure or be used by itself. It is important for you to understand there are two ways of dealing with reshaping the lower body:

- Limited or spot reduction, which is ideal for patients who have small, localized problem areas

- Large-area reduction, which is designed to treat larger areas such as the entire buttocks or both thighs

There are four methods of liposuction that can treat one or both types of reduction:

1. *Traditional liposuction* is a dry technique that simply suctions off the fat.

2. The *tumescent technique* consists of injecting a dilute solution of anesthetic into the area, causing the skin layer to balloon away so the fat is more easily targeted.

3. *UAL* (ultrasound-assisted liposuction) also relies on the tumescent injection, but after the cannula is inserted, a sonic laser pulse liquefies the fat, making it easier to remove.

4. *Lasers,* in some cases, are being adapted for use in liposuction as well. Because they cauterize— sear the flesh through heat—bleeding is minimized.

As described in Chapter 6, traditional liposuction is very straightforward. After making an incision and inserting the cannula, the doctor makes a jabbing motion that breaks up fat. Since there's no way to avoid tearing nerves and connective tissue, significant postoperative pain and swelling may occur. The yellow gelatinous fat and other fluids, including blood, are drawn through the tube by an external suction pump to a canister where it is eventually disposed of like all medical waste.

In the tumescent technique, the warmed tumescent liquid—a dilute solution containing lidocaine, epinephrine, and intravenous fluid—enters the fat, which becomes somewhat blanched. Liposuction is then performed on the tumesced areas. Although the technique can be used on any area of the body, it is commonly used on those lower-body areas that require enhanced precision, such as the inner thighs, knees, calves, and ankles. Another benefit: The expanded fat compartments allow the liposuction cannula to travel smoothly beneath the skin as the fat is removed. What used to be a bit of a "fat grab bag"—close your eyes and turn on the vacuums—has become a more precise harvest. Now, because the surgeon can more readily isolate the fat, there are at least three quantum advances of the tumescent approach that did not exist with traditional liposuction:

- Loss of blood and important body fluids is diminished.

- The underlying muscle and tissue are not so roughly pushed around.

- Patient recovery is often more speedy, with fewer lifestyle constraints, because there is less bruising and pain.

UAL and laser technology are being applied in conjunction with liposuction on the buttocks and other larger areas. Ultrasound waves liquefy the fat, making aspiration easier. The laser uses light energy to break up the fatty deposits and more readily separate them from tissue and muscles. Ultrasound technology, now with FDA approval, appears slightly ahead of laser technology in liposuction treatments. Both break up the fat so it is more easily suctioned. Advocates assert that this causes less bleeding and tissue damage, making recovery easier. And a steady stream of satisfied UAL patients bear out an improved recovery claim fairly consistently.

Endermologie: results without surgery

Endermologie, in some cases and with the right application, delivers some of the benefits of liposuction; however, it does not require invasive surgery. The sales brochure for Endermologie claims, "From head to toe, ENDERMOLOGIE enhances skin condition, and goes where no other available treatment can in combating fatty deposits that cause cellulite." The initial scuttlebutt suggests Endermologie, which was introduced in 1977, really does work. This technique claims to efficiently produce results with a nonsurgical procedure using electrical, heating pulses delivered through rollers that massage the cellulite. The treatment is applied during weekly sessions. A small, hand-held, boxlike contraption is placed on the treatment area. From this box, a large hose, much like that of a vacuum, connects to a master control instrument that resembles stripped-down professional dental equipment. The change is not immediate; treatments take up to 40 minutes and cost just under $100 each.

The before and after brochure photographs are fairly compelling, and the patented technique has been proven safe and effective. If the equipment were less costly, under $25,000 or so, there would be more opportunities for patients to explore results.

When prompted, most doctors agree they've heard positive feedback on the procedure. But many, including Dr. Paul Lorenc, claim the best results can be achieved when Endermologie is used as a follow up to liposuction. "I have noticed a truly good visible reduction in many patients. Arms and legs respond particularly well," says Dr. Lorenc. (Endermologie is discussed in more detail later in this chapter.)

Managing lower-body liposuction risks

Some prospects are not good candidates for lower-body surgery. Their weight may fluctuate considerably, they may be unlikely to follow recovery protocol, or their general health may present too many risk factors. If you're thinking about liposuction and are close to normal weight, two additional factors may make you a good prospect:

- You have fairly good skin tone.
- Your pockets of fat—considered to be smallish deposits—are in specific areas of the body that have proven to be resistant to diet and exercise.

Although many patients don't mirror this ideal, most experienced surgeons—on the record—feel a conservative approach to liposuction is the best. Liposuction must never be offered as a cure for or treatment of obesity. Obese patients are at risk because they can develop more complications, and their sedentary lifestyle, coupled with excess weight, places stress on the cardiovascular system. Off the record, a number of these same surgeons claim that overweight patients, truly obese candidates, over a series of treatments, can respond well to liposuction. Do they perform such treatments? Most say no, but a few actually do.

To manage your liposuction risk, you must realize that it is truly unrealistic to expect a new body; at most, liposuction can somewhat modify your contour.

One of the problems compounding liposuction risk today is that many patients pressure their surgeons into taking off more fat. Much like going to the service station for a simple oil change, once there, they ask for an engine overhaul. To minimize risk, never push for more surgery than your body can healthily accommodate.

How dermolipectomy helps the lower body bounce back

Dermolipectomy is a procedure that trims—or resects—the skin. As described in the previous chapter, incisions are made in skin folds, where they can be more easily camouflaged, and may be necessary to remedy drooping buttocks and flabby thighs and knees. For many procedures on the lower anatomy, dermolipectomy is usually considered ancillary to liposuction. However, with today's better and more refined techniques, liposuction alone may make your skin contract so that dermolipectomy will not be necessary.

Before you panic about the incisions, sutures, and scars, there is a variable worth putting into surgical perspective. While the notion of two operations at different times—instead of one with two procedures—may overwhelm you, explore your lifestyle. In many ways, some systems may be less traumatized by two *less invasive* procedures than by one extensive operation. By separating the two procedures—liposuction followed by skin resection— some patients find that their recuperation time is more comfortable and, surprisingly, they are able to

Watch Out!
If you have an endless supply of money, time and stamina, liposuction procedures over a few years may deliver significant changes. However, these dramatic results, evident in very overweight prospects, must be accompanied by exercise and healthy eating. And you may have to invest over one hundred thousand dollars if you desire perfection!

Unofficially...
The surgical procedure to resect excess, flaccid skin is sometimes also known as a *panniculectomy*. This procedure can be performed virtually anywhere on the body.

resume normal activity far sooner. This is one way to manage the stress liposuction can place on your recovery. Liposuction on the lower body can require a long time for some patients to bounce back. Discuss this possibility with your surgeon.

During the consultation with your surgeon, discuss the following surgical problems, though rare:

- Managing excessive fluid loss that can lead to shock
- Intervention for handling fluid, even blood accumulation, that may occur under the skin
- Skin rippling, crepiness, dimpling, or asymmetry that can persist after recovery
- Flap (or dog-ear) scarring
- Mottling of skin color

There are other issues to mull over in order to better manage surgical risk. Indeed, "death by liposuction"—despite a familiar Agatha Christie ring—is rare. However, after exploring some of the available data, unfortunate recent liposuction-related deaths do share several common denominators. They include:

- Liposuction surgery was extended over an unusually long period of time—up to nine hours or more.
- Significant areas of fat, perhaps unreasonable amounts, were treated.
- The treatment sought to accommodate more than three key areas.
- Healthy body fluids were not adequately managed throughout the procedures.
- Each patient's ability to rebound was compromised by fluid loss.

Here are a few findings of my own:

1. Serious complications and frightening risks pop up more frequently in nonhospital sites where the patient is treated for major, rather than minor, liposuction. Major surgery is always better served in a hospital setting.

2. These hideous scenarios are heightened when the surgeon leaves the site during the postoperative recovery period.

3. The patient's critical signs may not be monitored by a qualified staff member.

4. The staff member monitoring the patient's recovery is fully qualified and has the credentials; but, unfortunately, the person is not a full-time staff member. A full-time member brings an intuitive surgical sense to the critical postoperative period and knows what emergency help is available on-site.

You are the best candidate to explore the surgical site and get to know the doctor and staff, in order to determine if the support staff is capable of handling an emergency, notably yours.

If the surgery is small, why so much anesthetic?

Types of anesthetics can vary widely for lower-body liposuction. Another way to manage risk is to remind yourself that general anesthesia is best for major surgery. The amount of area to be treated and a person's own health play important roles. Be sure you understand the three possibilities:

1. If the area is small, typically local anesthetic is used; this is usually an injection of numbing anesthetic.

2. Local with sedation may be administered—by an IV—to induce sleep; this may be followed by

> 66
> Surgeons must be very careful When they take the knife! Underneath their fine incisions Stirs the Culprit—Life!
> —Emily Dickinson (1830–1886), No. 108
>

an injection of an anesthetic to numb the area being treated.

3. General anesthesia is induced by use of an anesthetic drug or gas, and a ventilator is required to assist breathing. This is reserved for more significant liposuction treatments.

In almost all liposuction operations, regardless of the chosen anesthetic, your doctor will use a local anesthetic with epinephrine, a vascular constrictor. This does two critically important things: It reduces bleeding during the operation and it aids in controlling postoperative pain.

Before agreeing to any procedure, understand the role of the anesthetic and be sure you agree with your surgeon's recommendation. And know who will monitor your response when you are essentially "out of it."

Common procedures

Liposuction can be performed on virtually any part of the body—the back, flanks, lower arms, love handles above the buttocks, and even within the tiniest of inner, upper thigh bulges.

Spot or local liposuction is used to treat small areas that do not respond to spot reduction exercises. You probably simply lack the genetic tools to change that area. One of the reasons, according to nutritionists and other medical experts, relates to our fat-cell count. The number of fat cells in the body is, as a rule, established by the time we become adolescents. These cells are durable, and, like balloons, have an amazing capacity to expand and store fat. Liposuction doesn't prick these balloons; instead, it removes them *permanently* from the area. When we're feeling too fat—not the weekend bloat

Unofficially...
Fat weighs little, relative to the space it occupies. A pound of fat takes up more room than a pound of muscle.

that passes by Tuesday—these cells are—simply put—inflated.

Common name: liposuction, buttock area

What it does: Removes excess flab from the fanny

Price range: $2,000 to $10,000

Operation duration: Limited liposuction can take 45 minutes to an hour. Standard liposuction takes one and a half to two hours.

Anesthetic: Typically local with sedation (MAC)

The procedure:

In buttock liposuction, a thin, hollow tube, or cannula, is inserted through one or more incisions, likely in the cheek fold; other incisions may be higher up. The area may have been treated with a tumescent liquid to cause the skin to balloon away from the fat and tissue. When a small, specific area is treated by limited liposuction, a small syringe is usually connected to the cannula to produce a vacuum. However, for standard liposuction, a larger and more powerful vacuum pump is used to treat larger areas. Many surgeons have designed their own cannulas—sleek, durable, yet delicate—to increase the aesthetic result. In UAL, the cannula is smaller than the one used in traditional liposuction.

In some patients, suctioning the fat could leave the fanny too flat and less than youthful looking. For these patients, a buttock lift repositions the fat in the upper buttock and rearranges the tissue of the cheek, making a natural, more appealing and rounded rear. This option should be discussed with your surgeon during the consultation.

Postoperative expectations:

It's likely you'll have incisions measuring three to six millimeters (there are 25.4 millimeters to the inch) where the cannula was inserted. Sutures may or may

Bright Idea
Aerobic exercise fuels circulation which borrows energy from fat cells, causing your weight to drop. You may have been trying to remove your bulges with the wrong exercise program. Explore such a possibility with a highly trained physical fitness pro.

not be used. Depending on the technique and amount of fat removed, it is likely that your pain will range from a throbbing discomfort to a more pronounced, unwelcome soreness, as if you sparred with a pro fighter who suddenly forgot your amateur status.

Keeping off your fanny will be necessary; make sure your surgeon advises you clearly about specific considerations for the recovery period. There's no getting around it, you'll ache. Any bruising and discoloration should disappear within 10 days or so. You can also expect swelling, which commonly peaks at three to four days and disappears within six weeks, sometimes longer. Some patients report numbness and a burning sensation at various intervals postoperatively with symptoms dissipating within four to six weeks.

An elastic bandage, support stockings, girdle, or special support garment is usually worn nearly continuously over the area for the first month. Final results, shown in the following photos, may not be evident for many months.

Moneysaver
Doctors recommend that patients with poor skin tone wear some type of support garment as much as possible for the month after the operation to reduce the possibility of skin dimpling, sagging, unevenness, or waviness. Ask your surgeon if tight Lycra bike shorts can be substituted if you want to look more fashionable during your recovery.

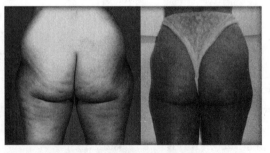

Before and after fanny liposuction results indicate a meaningful visual change. (Source: Dr. Gregory LaTrenta)

With your surgeon's approval, medical massage therapy—the type that equates to a lymphatic drainage massage therapy—may be tried in the second or third week after the operation. Many patients find this step provides relief for stiffness and sluggish circulation, thereby decreasing swelling.

Possible complications:

As with all procedures, the risk of infection, though typically low, must be carefully assessed. Blood clots can produce dangerous complications and some surgeons use blood thinners to offset this possibility. Also, losing too much fluid can lead to shock during the postoperative recovery period. Rare liposuction complications include pulmonary edema (the collection of fluid in the lungs), which can occur if too much fluid is administered; and lidocaine toxicity, which occurs if the solution's lidocaine content is too high. If general anesthetic is used, you will likely experience some queasiness since you can't sit up and eliminate "the whirlies." Not all liposuction treatments produce smooth, even results. And there are cases where scars stretch and pull and become more noticeable.

Although tumescent liposuction requires less anesthetic and also minimizes blood loss, patients undergoing the procedure still face the same risks and cosmetic complications associated with traditional liposuction surgery. Because blood loss is minimized during tumescent liposuction, use of the technique tends to reduce the chance that a blood transfusion will be needed.

Common name: fanny tuck

What it does: Reduces sagging in the buttocks and restores a more toned appearance

> 66
> Eating fresh pineapple or papaya during the postoperative period helps bruising disappear faster. The fruit has an enzyme that dissolves protein.
> —Timothy Callaghan, trained physical therapist, owner of Liberty Fitness
> 99

Price range: $4,500 to $9,000

Operation duration: Three hours or less

Anesthetic: Usually local

The procedure:

For best results, the patient should lose excess weight and remain at an ideal weight for three to six months before undergoing this procedure.

During the surgery, incisions are made in the fold of skin at the top of the legs. Long, wide, wedge-shaped strips of skin and fat, extending from the cheek crease to the sides of the hips, are cut off. The area is lifted and the incisions are closed. Many incisions are invisible to the eye following surgery, as the following photos show.

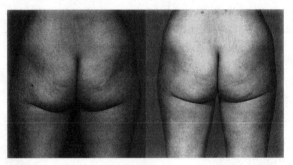

Before and after photos indicate satisfying shape and firm tone resulting from a fanny lift. (Source: Dr. Gregory LaTrenta)

To avoid damaging the incisions and the healing skin, you must avoid sitting for two or more weeks and may have to adjust your work schedule accordingly.

Postoperative expectations:

Pain and the inability to rest comfortably can make recovery seem tedious and endless. The amount of pain varies, but in several cases, the patients I interviewed said it was insignificant after the first week.

Swelling and bruising can also be a source of discomfort. People who typically sleep on their backs may find it difficult to rest comfortably.

Possible complications:

Hematomas can occur; these may resolve on their own or may need to be treated. Scars in the fold beneath the cheek, in some cases, never adequately disappear. For this aesthetic reason and because skin tone can lack firmness, the fanny lift often yields disappointing results. To offset this possibility, some surgeons feel an implant can deliver the correct solution. However, candidates must be chosen carefully and should be prepared for a lengthy recovery.

Common name: buttock implants

What it does: Rounds the upper buttocks for a more youthful appearance

Price range: $2,500 to $5,000

Operation duration: About one hour

Anesthetic: Local

The procedure:

To augment upper buttocks, semisolid silicone implants are inserted under the gluteus maximus muscle through an incision in the vertical cheek crease, just above the coccyx or tailbone. The implant—which is not the same ill-fated silicone implant used in breasts—is placed in a deep position to boost the muscle it seeks to enhance.

Postoperative expectations:

If the procedure is an adjunct to liposuction, many of the obvious expectations—bruising, swelling, and pain—will be magnified. Patients are unable to sit for several weeks or longer and many find discomfort—not to mention the inconvenience, pain, and drag associated with a more complicated

Moneysaver
Buttock implants can be combined with light liposuction of the thighs and saddlebags. If you're interested in having both procedures done at once, discuss it with your surgeon during the initial consultation, taking into account the cost, pain, and risks.

morning toilet routine—becomes a significant nuisance for a far longer time than anticipated.

Possible complications:

Again, complications that attend other implant procedures may also occur here: unnatural shape, movement, or dislocation of the implant, or, in rare cases, an unnaturally hard feeling and appearance to the buttock.

Common name: Endermologie

What it does: Delivers nonsurgical liposuction results over a series of treatments

Price range: $600 to several thousand dollars, depending on the area treated and number of treatments required

Operation duration: Each session lasts less than one hour

Anesthetic: None

The procedure:

Endermologie, through heat and deep and firm massage, works on the stagnant fluids in the subcutaneous tissue. Through repeated Endermologie applications, the flaccid, crepey appearance of the treated area becomes toned and more firm. While there is no medical term to define cellulite, its presence is often likened to the lumpiness of cottage cheese and Endermologie reduces this visible aspect.

An electric heating device is attached to the fatty area to be treated and is repeated over time—each series will vary—typically once or twice a week until results are obtained. You will be measured throughout the series to see if it is worth your continuing with treatments. The most successful results I have noted involve several women friends who simultaneously revamped their diets and exercise program while undergoing treatment. The results were excellent and I have a sense—though I can't prove it quantitatively—that Endermologie was a significant reducer of their cellulite.

Postoperative expectations: There is virtually no residual aftereffect.

Possible complications: None

Common name: thigh liposuction

What it does: Removes saddlebags and other bulges from the upper leg

Price range: $2,000 to $8,000

Operation duration: Varies according to area being worked on

Anesthetic: Varies according to area being worked on

The procedure:

Thigh liposuction is completely different from a thigh lift, described later in this chapter, which can be a very serious procedure.

In thigh liposuction, the cannula is manipulated between the muscle and fascia; the number of incisions may vary according to the surgeon and how much fat must be removed from where. If the bulges are on the inner thigh, typically an incision is made in the lower cheek crease to reduce fanny fat as well as inner thigh deposits. With the patient resting on her back, small incisions can be made to treat both inner and outer thigh fat pockets.

Postoperative expectations:

You will feel a significant amount of pain and will have to keep your feet elevated for at lest the first day, if not slightly longer, following the procedure. Your support girdle, a tight elastic bandage that you selected prior to your surgery, must be worn continuously for the next week and quite possibly longer. Once the major bruising and swelling has

Watch Out!
With traditional liposuction, it was once recommended that no more than one pound of fat be vacuumed. Now, with UAL, some surgeons claim a surprisingly large amount of fat— as much as 20 pounds or more—can be removed. However, many reputable surgeons strongly caution against this without a thorough evaluation of the patient first. Beware of ads that offer large amounts of fat removal.

vanished—up to four weeks or so—it's likely your doctor will recommend that you continue wearing the girdle.

An antibiotic ointment may be dispensed for daily treatment of the sutures until they are removed about a week later. Because your activity will be limited—and due to the anesthesia as well—you may become constipated. Be vigilant about eating a high-fiber diet, drink plenty of fluids (mostly water), and to minimize swelling, avoid salty and/or spicy foods. With liposuction only, you can remove your surgical garment to take a shower; the garment should be put back on immediately after drying off from the shower.

Do not drive until any medication you are taking wears off. Follow your doctor's protocol and resume easy walking, only, after a week or so. Do nothing strenuous until your doctor advises and if you feel a tweak of pain while moving around, don't repeat the action. In short, if anything hurts, don't do it!

Possible complications:

Lumpiness and unevenness, which may cause you concern at first, usually vanish over time. Make sure your incision sites are kept very clean. Be aware that internal bleeding is a possibility. Should you note an unusual spontaneous bruise, painful area, or a raised, swollen site, alert your doctor. You may need some touch-up liposuction to remove unevenness; in some cases a wiggle-shaped silhouette can result. Because wrinkling and rippling can occur, sometimes making cellulite appear worse, be aware that this long-term complication might develop.

Combining lipo for varied areas

Thigh liposuction is often done in tandem with liposuction for the buttocks. Because some women bear pockets of fat on the outer thighs that are closely embedded near the buttock area, surgeons often combine thigh and fanny liposuction procedures. Additionally, fatty ridges on the hip area can be diminished. Clearly, the cost and time variables change but often a more satisfying result is apparent.

The following photos show how the hips, outer and inner thighs, and buttock areas can be treated. Small incisions about a half inch or less, but sometimes slightly longer, will be made according to which area is to be treated. Be sure you understand during your consultation where the incisions will be placed. And because your amount of treatment will vary, you can expect to pay somewhere in the neighborhood of $5,000 and more simply for the surgeon's fee to have a multi-site, lower-body liposuction.

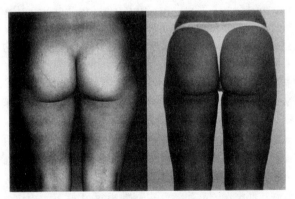

Several regions can be reduced, as these before and after photos show. The after photo illustrates how satisfying final results can be. In certain cases, liposuction can be combined over several areas in one procedure that can run from two to four hours. Costs vary widely—as do other issues—but surgical fees may average from $4,000 to $9,000. (Source: Dr. Gregory LaTrenta)

Common name: thigh lift

What it does: Raises a droopy upper leg to give a firmer, sometimes slimmer, contour

Price range: $5,000 to $10,000

Operation duration: Six hours or longer

Anesthetic: General

The procedure:

This surgery is demanding on the surgeon as well as the patient. Typically, the incision is made in the groin crease and continues around the inside of the thigh to the buttock crease. If both inner and outer thighs are being lifted, the incision often simply circles more of the leg. The skin is lifted off the underlying tissue and the flabby, excess skin is excised. The remaining skin is pulled up or lifted and sutured to the deep connective tissue of the thigh area and the groin. This deep suturing helps anchor the new shape. Temporary drains are inserted and the incisions are closed. This operation is considered a serious undertaking because the surgery can take as long as six hours or more, the incisions are significant, and your body is flipped several times during the procedure.

Postoperative expectations:

You will endure significant pain, which can be managed through prescriptions. Serious bruising, swelling, and discomfort from deeply imbedded sutures and the closing sutures are common. Drains are typically removed the following day. It's likely you'll stay in the hospital for a day after the procedure, perhaps longer. Your doctor will tailor a protocol for your recovery. Most patients find they are able to resume a light exercise program within eight weeks; shortly thereafter you may be operating at full speed.

Possible complications:

Internal bleeding can occur and should be carefully monitored. Blood clots, much like those that can occur after a tummy tuck, are also possible, though the reported incidence is slightly higher with this surgery. Discuss blood thinners and preventative measures with your surgeon before agreeing to undergo this significant surgery.

Common name: calf buffing, calf implants

What it does: Adds shape to lower legs

Price range: $2,000 to $4,000

Operation duration: 45 minutes or longer

Anesthetic: Local

The procedure:

Working through incisions in the fold behind the knees, the surgeon positions implants on either or both sides of the calf to enhance thinly defined legs. The implants are placed deep within the dense fascia. The incisions must be taped for one and one-half months.

Body builders, unable to gain the bulk and volume they desire through diet and exercise, often seek calf implants. And the procedure, when used on women, may also be performed in tandem with liposuction of the ankles and knees.

Postoperative expectations:

With implants, the standard expectations apply: pain, swelling, bruising, and discomfort. Infection possibilities must be carefully monitored and bending your leg must be avoided for at least several days. Keep your legs elevated and apply iced compresses for the first two days.

Possible complications:

Associated implant complications include possible unnatural shape, dislocation, or movement of the

implant, and general dissatisfaction with the resulting correction.

Just the facts

- Lower-body liposuction is serious; find the most
  qualified surgeon you can and remain active in
  the decision process.

- Understand who will manage your postoperative recovery immediately after surgery; determine if that person is qualified and is a full-time
  employee.

- Don't pressure your surgeon into considering
  more fat removal than he or she suggests in your
  consultation.

- Fully understand and evaluate all that recovery
  requires; can you afford the time and the
  expense, endure the pain, and observe the strict
  protocol?

How the skin heals ▪ Procedures for
making scars less noticeable ▪
The latest on lasers ▪ Treating varicose and
spider veins ▪ Bye-bye birthmarks, neckline
sun damage, and other skin irregularities

Skin Corrections

Chapter 14

By examining a few basics on skin and how the skin heals, you can see why your dermis plays such a critical role in all cosmetic surgery procedures. Cosmetic surgery—apart from correcting facial features, recontouring your body, or rejuvenating your appearance—can now treat many large areas of skin such as your back or neckline.

Many of these large area treatments involve state-of-the-art technology. The great leap, in part, is due to the application of lasers. This chapter explains the differences between the key laser types and how they are used in certain procedures.

If you are troubled by patches of facial scarring, moles, ugly skin tags, brown spots, or even a birthmark, sometimes called a port wine stain, there are a variety of ways to diminish each, as you'll discover in this chapter. Or maybe you're tired of that "branding iron" sun damage that races all over your neckline and chest. You can lose the superficial signs of that baked-in sun damage and still have money left over to buy a new off-the-shoulder dress.

Unless, of course, you're a guy; in that case, get out your Bermuda reds and celebrate!

Everything you care to know about scars

Even if you've managed to get through life without a single scar, read this section. By grasping a few basics on scarring, you'll better understand how most methodologies for skin treatment actually work.

One of the more challenging, everyday hurdles for a plastic surgeon is making a scar less obvious. For some reason, we average folk are convinced that plastic surgeons are magicians. They actually can make a scar vanish. Ironically, what cosmetic surgeons often do is a form of magic—they create an illusion to improve an aspect or help disguise the imperfection.

In truth, a scar can never be completely erased, but it can usually be improved.

Remember that old adage: Time heals all wounds? Well, there is much truth to that when it comes to skin in general. Many scars diminish over time. Nevertheless, when it comes to cosmetic surgery scars, most patients believe that early intervention will improve the problem. But in fact, the best strategy is to do nothing for a while.

Here's why that strategy is best.

Scars are made of collagen, connective tissue composed of protein that is found throughout the body. During wound healing, the cut area (even if it is sutured) produces more collagen than normal. Blood vessels—alerted that there is a wound—also increase in size as they bring nourishment to the wounded area. The scar becomes prominent and red. Then, at some point, the collagen usually begins to break down as the wound heals, and the

> "
> One writes of scars healed, a loose parallel to the pathology of the skin, but there is no such thing in the life of an individual. There are open wounds, shrunk sometimes to the size of a pinprick, but wounds still.
> —*Tender Is the Night*, F. Scott Fitzgerald, 1896–1940
> "

blood vessels decrease in size. This is what causes the scar to fade, soften, and sometimes flatten.

The final appearance of a scar can take more than a year to mature. Certain areas of the body are more likely to produce wider, thicker scars, especially where the skin is pulled and stretched. (If you're in doubt, check your knees.)

So, apart from the depth of the wound, the inten-sity of a scar depends on the location and the person's own ability to heal. Some people form thin and pale scars; others produce thicker scars. People with dark skin are more prone to form keloid scars—the kind that are thick, raised, sometimes shiny. (Chapter 10 explains keloids.)

If you grasp this healing process, you can appreciate why certain procedures—as you read through them in the following sections—are best accomplished over a series of smaller steps interspersed with time for healing. The surgeon treats the skin but, more often than not, the skin responds in slow motion.

There are various ways to alter a scar so it becomes less noticeable. Steroid treatments typically retard collagen buildup. Some scars can also be surgically altered to remove the most noticeable area. Surgery to remove a scar can be as simple as cutting away the scar and sewing the skin back together in such a way that the incision heals better. Or sanding a pebbly, raised scar with a dermabrader can tone it down to the level of the surrounding skin. One red flag: There is a limit to the amount of dermabrasion that can be done repeatedly in one area.

Sometimes little balloons—called *tissue expanders* or *new skin balloons*—are placed beneath pristine skin near the scar. The balloons are then filled with a saline solution. When the fresh skin has been

Watch Out!
Many scars are poor candidates for revision, and in some cases the procedures done to diminish the scars make the situation worse.

adequately stretched—over weeks and months—the balloons are taken out. The scarred skin can be cut off and the balloon-stretched skin pulled over the previously scarred area, much like a form of human reupholstery.

Every scar revision must be tailored to the individual. A common desire is to treat the entire scar at one time, much the way some liposuction patients want their whole body treated at once. For large scars, this is not recommended. Instead, a series of intermediary revisions typically give more predictable—and satisfactory—results.

The two most common complaints about scars are irregularities of contour—whether the scar is sunken or raised, wide or thick—and color flaws. The most common scars tend to fall into one of these three categories:

- *Sunken scars.* Sometimes ironically known as depressed scars, these sunken lines or patches are often characterized by a widening bevel—as if a grooved chisel was used—which is due to insufficient tissue. Revision frequently involves advancing healthy skin over the depressed area and suturing the area carefully with fine stitches.

- *Raised scars.* The opposite of a depressed scar is one with *too* much tissue. The scar sits up high. Revision involves resecting the excess scar tissue, then replacing it with the adjoining healthy skin. Raised scars may also be treated with a variety of chemical peels, dermabrasion, and certain lasers. Some surgeons or dermatologists use a combination of several methodologies, deployed in various parts of the scar.

- *Thick scars.* Keloid scars are the third most common. In some cases, direct excision works best to improve the appearance of these scars. Initial treatment of any thick scar may also involve injections of medications containing steroids to soften and flatten the scar while stopping production of additional scar tissue. Both of these approaches may also use a tight dressing or garment that flattens the scar.

Common name: z-plasty or w-plasty scar revision

What it does: Reshapes a more complex scar, making it less obvious

Price range: $500 and up, depending on size and complexity

Operation duration: Less than half an hour for small scars; under one hour for most other scars

Anesthetic: Local

The procedure:

Simple scar revision follows the direction or integrity of the scar. More complex scars may demand a different direction. There is w-plasty, in which the surgeon makes a w-shaped incision over the scar. Z-plasty calls for a z-shaped incision through the scar.

The remaining triangular-shaped flaps of skin, top and bottom, reverse the direction of the scar, forming a backward "z." Existing scar tissue is excised and a new, less obvious scar remains, though its overall length is longer.

Postoperative expectations:

There is little discomfort associated with most average scar revisions. However, perfect skin hygiene is necessary. Your doctor will prescribe the appropriate protocol that may include medicinal ointments, antibiotics, or a mild over-the-counter painkiller if the scar throbs during the early healing process. Give the revision time—many months—to heal.

Possible complications:
There are few, if any, complications, though in some cases, the revised scar may not appear much improved. Again, give the area a lot of time to heal. Be sure your surgeon or dermatologist can properly evaluate how the scar is likely to react to revision. Choose the most qualified doctor you can to revise the scar.

Common name: acne scar treatment

What it does: Reduces the pockmarks and creasing due to acne

Price range: $400 to $2,000, depending on the area treated

Operation duration: Varies, depending on the type of treatment and size of the area

Anesthetic: Local

The procedure:

Ice pick scars often extend through the upper dermis into the deeper dermis or fat tissue. This is what makes them obvious to the eye, and it is also why the scars are tough to eradicate. In fact, completely ridding the skin of acne scars really can't be done effectively. However, there are some solid breakthroughs that deliver better results than the former options of chemosurgery, injectable fillers, and punch grafting. (Collagen injections, if effective, deliver only temporary results; if not effective, results may make the lesions look even bigger.)

First, depending on the number of ice pick scars and their proximity to each other, some surgeons might excise up to eight lesions at a time, suture each with a tiny stitch, and allow this cluster to heal over a period of eight weeks or longer. Thereafter, laser resurfacing with the high-energy CO_2 laser has proven to be a more effective remedy for *atrophic scars*—those that dip into the skin— than for *hypertrophic scars*—those that are raised. Atrophic scars also respond to dermabrasion, especially if they are remedied first by excision and closure. Following a suitable healing time, skin around the pitted areas is abraded to a lower level, producing a more even appearance.

Sutured scars that are close together can heal poorly, creating the appearance of a gap once the sutures are removed. The area can be numbed by injection or by freezing the skin with a refrigerant. In addition to inducing anesthesia, freezing the skin with a refrigerant can also make the skin firmer, helping the surgeon deliver a uniform abrasion.

If a large area is to be treated, laser or dermabrasion may be performed in small units to ensure a uniform skin removal. Bleeding that attends dermabrading (but not laser resurfacing) is controlled by pressure, and an occlusive gauze dressing is often applied.

Postoperative expectations:

There will be intense swelling, oozing, and crusting over the treated area. With dermabrasion, as the gauze begins to spontaneously separate within three to five days, you may be told to cover the healing area with ointment. Ice compresses will help control discomfort for the first few days; these should be cloth-wrapped and not wet. Keep your head elevated. If you notice milia, small whiteheads that may be exacerbated by the ointment, alert your doctor. Around the fourth or fifth day, you should be able to wash the area with a mild, soap-free cleanser. If this hurts, wait a day. When cleansing or removing make-up in the future, never rub your skin in a rough manner. Blot it dry; never scrub.

Watch Out!
If you had radiation treatments for acne when you were younger, alert your doctor. This could put you at increased risk for worse scarring. This is also true for any treatment with the oral anti-acne drug isotretinoin (Accutane); again, alert your doctor. You may have to wait for the medicine to leave your system.

As with z-plasty or w-plasty scar revision, the healing area will appear intensely red, resembling a sunburn, and can become crusty and flaky. This resolves over a period of time that is highly individualized. In some cases, a tender redness is prolonged for months, particularly if the patient exposes herself to the sun. In other cases, the patient appears normal within several weeks to a month, depending on how deep the abrasion is and the nature of her complexion.

Possible complications:

In rare cases, an infection can form but is usually easily treated with a topical antibiotic.

Treating unsightly veins

As we age, veins on ankles, legs, and backs of hands become more apparent as muscle mass, tissue, and fat deposits begin to diminish. These veins are healthy and should not be treated. Instead, this section deals with irregularities that can detract from appearance and, in some cases, create discomfort. *Phlebology* is the study and treatment of veins which, for cosmetic treatment, tend to show up near the surface of skin in two basic forms:

1. Bulging, larger varicose veins

2. Smaller, wispier spider veins

Various procedures can be done to soften the appearance or even eliminate irregular veins. Unfortunately, prospective patients are often confused by the quickly emerging treatment methodologies. Which approach is the best? Truthfully, there are many excellent ways to treat a vein. Exactly which methodology depends on the doctor; your physician pretty much makes the selection based on his or her expertise.

Since the advent of lasers, this methodology represents a growing and vital treatment. It's important to appreciate how different lasers work. There are many types of lasers. Dermatologists and plastic surgeons often have several laser systems, each of which can be very expensive. In order to get a doctor to purchase a laser system, manufacturers often try to pitch the five or more treatments *one* laser can deliver. But, for the most part, you'll find that physicians claim that each laser does only one treatment the best; the secondary uses are usually inferior. The most popular lasers, which use short bursts (or pulsed waves), are shown in the following table.

Type of Laser	What It's Used For
CO_2 (with pattern generator to save time)	Skin resurfacing to correct problems such as sun damage and indented scars
Q-switched Alexandrite	Removing tattoos and bluish skin imperfections
Q-switched ruby	Removing signs of aging, sun spots, freckles, and brown age spots
Flashlamp-pulsed-dye	Removing red birthmarks, diluted capillaries, rosacea, sun damage, spider veins, some scars

A number of the older lasers use a continuous wave and are preferred by some skin specialists. These include:

Type of Laser	What It's Used For
CO_2 continuous wave	Some eyelid operations and incisions
Argon	Removing large, resistant vessels or nodules in port wine stains
Copper bromide, copper vapor, or krypton	Removing small vascular lesions called cherry angiomas or larger spider veins

It is wise to select the surgeon based on his or her capability, and then go with the methodology and equipment that the doctor recommends. As explained in earlier chapters, choosing a methodology first and then seeking a doctor who uses that methodology is a limited approach to finding the best remedy for your situation.

Varicose veins

Large, bulging veins known as *varicose veins* can be caused by heredity, disease, hormonal changes, even pregnancy. They can cause discomfort, pain, burning, and itching sensations and can lead to phlebitis or ulceration. Essentially, valves in the vein prevent the flow of blood that has circulated to the feet to return upward to the heart. This pressure causes the vein to balloon or become irregular. Varicose veins usually occur on the inner lower part of the leg, and less often on the back of the leg.

Unofficially...
Venography is a technique for viewing the interior of a vein by injecting a solution that is visible on X-ray; passage of the fluid through the vein can be recorded in a series of pictures called a *venogram*.

If you have large varicose veins, discuss options for treating them with your doctor. He or she may recommend vein stripping, which is the actual surgical removal of the vein; injection, which I discuss next; or some other option. No matter which treatment is used to banish varicose veins, invariably, like blue phantoms, some recur. The return may be a smaller version of the previous vein, or one that is virtually imperceptible.

Common name: vein injection (sclerotherapy)

What it does: Diminishes the appearance of varicose veins and larger spider veins

Price range: Up to $300 per injection

Operation duration: From 15 minutes to one hour or more, depending on the size and number of veins

Anesthetic: None

The procedure:

Sclerotherapy involves injecting veins with an irritating solution called a sclerosing agent, which causes inflammation and a clot to form in the vein, stopping blood flow. (Note that this is not the dangerous deep vein clot that may travel to the lungs, causing a pulmonary embolism.) For someone with a lot of leg veins, three to six visits are usually required. Your legs may be photographed for your medical records.

With the patient resting on the examination table, the skin over the veins is cleaned with an antiseptic solution. Using one hand to stretch the skin taut, the doctor (or nurse) injects either saline or a chemical solution (called a sclerosing agent) into the vein. Bright, indirect light and magnification help ensure that the process is completed with maximum precision. The patient feels a prick of the needle followed by a slight burning sensation that soon vanishes. The sclerosing agent causes inflammation within the veins and they collapse. The compressed vein wall seals itself and the vein is closed. Approximately one injection is administered for every inch of vein—anywhere from 5 to 40 injections per treatment session.

After treatment, the area is wrapped in a compressed bandage to keep possible swelling and redness to a minimum, and the patient is sent home. Avoiding aspirin or alcohol for two weeks before the procedure is wise to prevent heavy bleeding during the operation.

Postoperative expectations:

The bandage is removed after about five days. The patient can bathe during that time but care must be taken to keep the bandage dry. Depending on the

Timesaver
It's important to stay out of the sun for about a month after sclerotherapy, or you could end up with blotchy patches—the result of iron pigments from blood trapped inside the collapsed vein. They always go away, but it can take a long time. To be safe, consider scheduling your sclerotherapy during the winter months.

type of solution that was used, some itching may be experienced along the vein route. This itching should fade after a day or two. There may be some bruising, which will heal within a week. Some discoloration within the veins can occur; this normally fades in the following weeks and months. Regular activities can resume during the healing, although heavy exercise should be put off for two or three days. Aerobic exercise, even walking, may aid in the healing and prevention of varicose veins. The corrective procedure may also remedy related symptoms including aching, burning, swelling, and night cramps. Compression stockings may need to be worn for two to three weeks.

Possible complications:

Because saline is salt water, a naturally occurring body fluid, there is little chance of an allergic reaction, though in some cases there's a mild swelling. There may be prolonged skin discoloration. The treatment is not always successful and several treatments are often necessary to obtain the desired result and to clear more difficult areas.

Spider veins

Millions of women are bothered by spider veins—those small yet unsightly clusters of red, blue, or purple veins that most commonly appear on the thighs, calves, and ankles. (Men may also have spider veins—but their appearance isn't usually as troubling to men as it is to women.) It's estimated that at least half of the adult female population has spider veins. The same lasers used to rejuvenate the face can also treat unsightly spider veins, which are the result of heredity, pregnancy, hormonal shifts, weight gain, sitting or standing too long, or certain medications.

Known in the medical world as *telangiectasias* or *sunburst varicosities,* spider veins lie close to the surface of the skin. Although these super-fine veins connect to the large vein system, they are not an essential part of it. Most spider veins radiate from a central point like a pinwheel or they branch out like a little tree. Other spider veins are simple lines, nearly straight, with no wispy trails bursting outward; these are commonly seen on the inner knee. Pinwheel types cluster on the outer thighs.

Common name: spider vein removal (laser)

What it does: Destroys the small network of vessels that can mar the skin

Price range: $200 and up, depending on methodology and area

Operation duration: Depends on the area treated, but generally less than 15 minutes

Anesthetic: None

The procedure:

The flashlamp-pulsed-dye laser helps take care of smaller spider veins and broken capillaries on the face. It blocks off the blood flow and collapses the veins by producing short bursts of energy that target specific skin colors (in this case, red), but doesn't affect the surrounding dermis. One or two laser sessions may be required.

Postoperative expectations:

Lasers may produce purple blemishes, which will disappear. Ice compresses will help manage any mild swelling. In some cases, there may be some residual brownish pigmentation; this may take days or weeks to fade.

Possible complications:

Complications are rare, but veins may not totally respond to treatment and may recur.

Common name: permanent make-up

What it does: Adds permanent color—such as brown to the eyebrow area—to enhance or restore natural pigmentation that may have been lost

Price range: $200 to $2,000

Operation duration: Depending on the area, about one hour or less

Anesthetic: None, or mild numbing agent

The procedure:

Permanent make-up is applied by injecting pigmentation into the bottom layer of the skin, called the "dermis," much like a tattoo is applied. The procedure can deliver permanent coloring to the eye area in the form of eyebrow liner, eye shadow, and/or eyeliner; to the lips in the form of lipstick and/or lip liner; or to the skin in the form of blush. It can also be used to restore color to an area of skin that has lost its natural color, such as an injury to the lips.

Permanent make-up is not taught in medical schools and some states restrict who can offer the process. Although it is done by some cosmetic surgeons, it's most commonly performed by a dermatologist or aesthetician in a salon.

Postoperative expectations:

Unless this procedure is done by a fully qualified doctor or top-notch beauty aesthetician, your results may be much like having a friend pierce your ears: infection, incorrect placement, and throbbing pain. If you select a doctor, be sure he or she is experienced in performing this procedure and that you both share similar tastes. If not, the color may be too harsh or fake looking. Look for a doctor or practitioner who has a conservative approach and who will perform the procedure under the most pristine and antiseptic conditions.

Watch Out!
Permanent make-up training is highly inconsistent and no special license is needed! Training can consist of a two-day seminar or simply viewing an instructional videotape. Any person who has the equipment can be in business as soon as they find a paying customer. Shop wisely and ask to *see* and *speak* to satisfied customers.

Possible complications:

While the skin and human body work miracles in order to heal, an infection that accompanies a permanent-make-up procedure can rupture the skin and totally compromise results. You may have to resort to dermabrasion or laser resurfacing to restore the treated area, which may never look the same. Reduce the chance of infection by keeping the area scrupulously clean.

Common name: tattoo removal

What it does: Eradicates or diminishes decorative tattoos

Price range: $300 to $1,500

Operation duration: Less than one hour

Anesthetic: Local

The procedure:

A Professional tattoo is made by repeatedly pricking the skin with a needle loaded with pigment. The needle deposits the color close to the outer layer of the skin, giving a crisp outline and sharp color.

There are several ways to remove tattoos surgically. Dermabrasion can remove the superficial pigmentation. Small tattoos can be surgically excised and resutured with excellent results. Larger tattoos must be excised and closed with a local flap or a skin graft. The use of flaps has recently been aided by tissue expansion techniques. Both flaps and grafts result in new skin and complete tattoo removal, with only a small scar remaining.

When tattoos are removed by laser therapy, the technique is somewhat different. Currently, the CO_2 laser is used for tattoo removal. It produces intense light of a specific wave length, sharply focused, which destroys tissue. While the tattoo itself may not be removed, the new skin masks the imbedded color.

Watch Out!
Amateur tattoos may be deeper in the layers of the skin or even below the skin in the subcutaneous fatty tissue. Such tattoos appear somewhat muted and blurred, in contrast to those professionally applied, and they are often more difficult to remove.

Postoperative expectations:
There may be swelling and bruising following dermabrasion or excision.

Possible complications:
With dermabrasion or excision there is a chance of infection, which can be prevented by keeping the area antiseptically clean. In CO_2 resurfacing, the new scar formation can also be of poor quality and may not mature to a normal skin color.

Common name: removal of birth marks (port wine stains)

What it does: Diminishes or removes uneven pink or purple skin irregularities

Price range: $700 for small marks, $2,000 for large facial or limb marks; given as a series, each individual treatment may average $300

Operation duration: Usually less than one hour to accommodate treating only small portions at a time

Anesthetic: Mild local if needed

The procedure:
Some people don't mind unevenly colored skin patches; they view them with affection, much like a rare tattoo. Others opt to remove the odd patch.

The most common and successful way to fade port wine stains is by using a laser that emits microsecond-long pulses of yellow light, destroying the blood vessels that create the blotch of red. These birth marks represent a dense web of tangled blood vessels just below the surface of the skin. They may darken with age and develop a lumpy texture with small bumps or nodules; these are blood vessels that can bleed excessively when cut. Only very small sections can be treated at one time, so a series of treatments may have to be extended over many months, even years.

Postoperative expectations:

Minor redness and swelling fades within 48 hours and the skin feels sunburned. The bluish debris under the skin will disappear in 10 days or so as the circulatory system cleans the area. Don't panic if the treated area looks as red as before; this will fade over the next few weeks. After several weeks, the results should be more dramatic.

Possible complications:

Because very small areas are treated in each session, there are few complications when the procedure is performed conservatively and correctly. But lasers are extremely powerful instruments. Because the skin can be overtreated, choose an expert who has a lot of experience in removing port wine stains or birthmarks.

Common name: body peels

What it does: Removes sun damage from the back, neckline, chest, arms, or hands

Price range: $750 and up, depending on the area to be treated

Operation duration: Less than one hour; a series of treatments is usually required

Anesthetic: Local if needed and depending on chemical used

The procedure:

Glycolic lotions with more concentrated AHA (alpha-hydroxy acid) of 50 to 70 percent can be used to treat greater skin areas that may be marred by acne scars, age spots, or sun damage.

Treatment usually requires at least eight peels to alleviate significant damage, and these are scheduled over time, a couple of weeks apart, even longer. For more serious damage, as many as twelve peels may be required to normalize the appearance.

Unofficially...
The younger the patient, the easier it may be to effectively treat the port wine stain.

In some cases, Retin-A, dispensed by a dermatologist, can reduce the appearance of stretch marks. While Retin-A penetrates deeper than over-the-counter alpha-hydroxyl acid peels, results take longer. This treatment, however, should be carefully monitored by a dermatologist or plastic surgeon since the patient can frequently apply too much in an attempt to hasten the correction. Delivering too much Retin-A to the site can create an uncomfortable skin irritation that works against the problem the patient is seeking to remedy.

Postoperative expectations:

Depending on the depth of the peel, the newly regenerating skin appears thinner and more delicate, and either very red or very pink. With all peels, except very mild glycolic solutions, a significant scaly crust forms and falls off, though afterward no treatment is necessary other than frequent gentle washing and application of a bland ointment to help retain skin moisture. With deep and medium peels, ointments containing cortisone-like agents are sometimes prescribed.

All exposure to the sun must be carefully avoided for three to six months. It's best to avoid the sun altogether or use a strong sun block.

Possible complications:

Problems, from minor to severe, usually relate to uneven skin pigmentation results. In some cases, this may be due to the unpredictability of your skin type and may be beyond the direct control of the surgeon. Some patients develop a noticeable line of demarcation between the treated and untreated skin area. Make sure you discuss this possibility with your doctor before you agree to a peel. Occasionally, areas of splotchy hyperpigmentation develop after a chemical peel. Again, this problem occurs most frequently in people with dark complexions, but may also occur in light-skinned patients after sun exposure. Repeeling may be necessary to correct this, but it may have to be delayed long after the first peel. Pigmented facial blemishes present before the peel are frequently relatively darker after the procedure.

Just the facts

- How skin responds is highly individual; disappointing results may be unavoidable and will vary according to methodology and the imperfection being treated.

- All skin healing requires a great deal of time; be willing to wait for results before you seek corrective procedures.

- Be sure the laser procedure your doctor suggests has been sufficiently developed and tested.

- Follow skin care protocol diligently.

Postoperative Survival Guide

GET THE SCOOP ON...
Managing your wounds after surgery ▪ Understanding that swelling and bruising are normal
after-effects of surgery ▪ Taking control of your
healing: nutrition, elevation, and other tips

PART VI

Managing the Healing Process

Chapter 15

The patient has two very specific needs—
keeping the wound process moving along
and maintaining good nutrition—that must
be effectively managed after surgery. These two
considerations take on added significance after any
hospital stay but are essential to a good recovery
following cosmetic surgery. This chapter gives you
the inside information you'll need to rate whether
your individual response is on track.

Following surgery, you may feel a complete sense
of physical and emotional disarray; you're totally
overwhelmed. While this is normal, anything that
you can do prior to your coming home will help
your wound and recovery process enormously. (I'll
give you some additional tips for at-home care in the
next chapter.) If you've never had stitches before or
haven't had to treat a significant wound, be sure to
ask your surgeon and the supervising staff what you
can expect and write down their suggestions. The
most important thing to remember is to keep your

hands away from the treated area. As you examine your sutures and the crisping of natural liquids that may be oozing, you may think washing the area with a little warm sudsy water will help. Don't!

This chapter takes you through the internal process your body initiates in order to heal itself and speed recovery. It shows you how you can take responsibility, too. The surgeon may perform the procedure and then stitch you up, but you're really on your own once you arrive home. By grasping wound management, you'll learn how to protect the surgeon's handiwork.

Effective wound management

Wounds heal by *epithelialization,* a fancy word that simply means that skin cells spread out, creating a sealed, protective cover over the wound. The process also includes *collagen formation* (the formation of scar tissue over the wound) and *scar remodeling* (the phases a scar goes through). Scarring is anticipated after most operations, but the amount of noticeable scarring can be minimized by the practiced skill and extensive experience of proven surgical techniques. Your role in wound management is significant; proper healing depends largely on how strictly you follow your doctor's protocol.

There are basically two types of wounds: *closed wounds* and *open wounds.* Let's take a closer look at each.

Closed wounds

A closed wound is the usual sutured incision, such as the suturing of the cut line near the front of the ear following the undermining, lifting, and excision of tissue, at the end of a face lift. The entire face-lift incision both in front and behind the ear will be closed with sutures.

Healing begins at the time of the skin's injury. There is local accumulation of specific cells and naturally produced chemical substances. As these liquids rush in, swelling or edema occurs. This is good! Without this wash of natural liquids, healing cannot succeed. Swelling reaches its greatest range within two or three days and then begins to diminish. That's why treating the area with cold compresses is so critical during the early period. It keeps excessive swelling at bay.

After about five days, a type of cell called the *fibroblast* begins to deposit a complicated protein molecule called *collagen*. Collagen is the basic protein in the lower layers of normal skin. Equally important, it is the substance that we clinically identify as the scar. The collagen accumulation—an effective systemic storage warehouse process—continues for approximately four to six weeks after wound healing begins. Collagen production then reaches a maximum level. This is usually dictated by your own healing schedule and the maximum support that the skin requires in that area. This is why scars can look worse in certain areas—hands may not heal well because fingers—in fact the entire hand—must be flexible. More collagen may be produced at all joints, imparting a thicker scar appearance. Eventually, though, collagen production ebbs as the healing wound reaches its optimum strength.

If you break protocol when the scar is vulnerable—and each person is different—you may undo the best handiwork your surgeon has contributed to the overall results. This is why your surgeon's protocol likely will dictate:

Watch Out!
Some swelling is perfectly natural; without it, wound healing will not proceed normally. It is best managed by repeatedly applying cold compresses— 20 minutes on, 20 minutes off— for the first day or so after surgery. However, excessive angry red swelling that pulls at sutures and stretches the skin is a sign of infection and is *not* normal; contact your doctor immediately.

- No strenuous activity
- No elevating your blood pressure (via sex or bending)
- No "breaking a sweat"

After this six-week period, scarring begins to change. The incision, somewhat elevated because of the collagen supply, may also appear a bit red because of the concentration of a new local blood vessel and blood supply. As the scar adjusts, the puffiness or elevation flattens. Ultimately a pale, skin-colored, flat line remains.

This phase of fading and flattening, called *scar maturation,* may require a full year or more after wound healing begins. Because collagen slightly reconfigures itself, most scars will contract in length during maturation. While this is beneficial in most areas, it can be unfavorable when a scar is placed too near a joint—liposuction of the inner knee, for example. As the scar contracts, the incision can feel too tight. Invariably the skin adjusts or you'll simply become accustomed to the "pull," which should dissipate over time.

Open wounds

In some cosmetic procedures (smokers suffer more), infection can occur and the wound must be cleaned, cutting the dead skin away. Popping a suture or causing bleeding may lead to infection. These are two examples of open wounds, and, though rare, understanding what is required to get healing underway again may encourage you to take fastidious care and follow your surgeon's protocol.

There are three variables that mark an open wound:

1. Virtually all open wounds are contaminated.

2. The protective skin cover is missing; it's pulled off and away.

3. Open wounds experience *wound edge contraction,* meaning the edges seek to close themselves off and heal the open patch.

A few days after a major open wound occurs, a very bright red, granular-looking soft scab, called *granulation tissue,* forms at the base of the wound. This tissue consists of many small, new blood vessels and *myofibroblasts,* special healing cells. This new collection of vessels acts as a kind of plumbing system, dedicated to keeping the area clean and carrying away debris that might cause infection. At this time, your body's own natural defense mechanism, including the presence of white blood cells, attacks bacteria and keeps infection from invading your wound.

Like fibroblasts, myofibroblasts can also deposit collagen. However, this collagen is remarkably pliant, almost double-jointed, meaning it has the ability to shrink or contract. Thus, these cells gradually pull the edges of an open wound toward the center, producing more scar tissue as the contraction proceeds.

Depending on wound size, over a period of days to weeks, the wound draws together and shrinks to a small size, eventually closing like an evaporating puddle of water. The ends are bridged by new growing epithelial cells from the margins of the existing skin.

In addition to creating pockets of collagen, remodeling the scar, and contracting the wound edge, epithelial cells seal the skin wound. This may follow quickly, perhaps within 24 hours after careful suturing of an open wound.

The epithelial cells keep fluids within the body and bacteria and dirt out. So speedy is this process that many cosmetic surgery dressings can be

Unofficially...
Open wounds may yield a scar that is surprisingly small because of the progressive contraction of the wound edges. However, in cosmetic surgery, open wounds must be avoided at all costs, because even a small open wound produces a visible scar.

removed after the first or second day. By then the wound has been sealed and is contained by its own normal cellular membrane. The scholar Celus first identified the four characteristics of abnormal wound activity about 2,000 years ago. These four cardinal signs indicate an infection:

1. Pain

2. Swelling

3. Warmth or heat

4. Redness

Bright Idea
To save yourself hours of unnecessary worry, write the following note on an index card and carry it with you for one year after surgery: "A scar is most noticeable at six weeks, due to elevation and redness. The ultimate, fine, mature, pale scar takes at least one year to mature. I will not entertain scar revision until 12 months or more after surgery."

Scars and healing

In the rare case of having to have your suture or wound opened, do expect your surgeon to align the tissues accurately so the scar will be well concealed and as thin as possible. Ask where the scar is likely to form and how it may look. Remember, practically all cosmetic surgery involves scarring; but for many operations, such as a face lift, the scars are so small that they are almost invisible. Also, an expert surgeon knows scars can be hidden in areas where, for the most part, they remain concealed. But you must wait at least a year before you evaluate how well your scars have healed. It cannot be emphasized enough that all skin wounds heal with scar tissue. Regardless of how carefully wounds are closed, some visible scarring is likely.

Plastic surgeons depend on normal scar formation for healing. They tend to be concerned about concealing normal scars in natural folds and shadows. You, however, can share this burden by realistically discussing incisions and any alternatives that the surgeon can offer, should you worry about the line being very obvious. Undertake this scar exploration several weeks prior to your surgery.

If you are extremely sensitive about scar incisions on your face, do what one patient did to diffuse the issue. She spent a day with her imaginary scar. Here's how you can do it, too:

■ With a washable-ink, felt-tip pen, draw a thin line on your face where the scar will be.

■ Go through the day and see if people notice it. How many of these people are you likely to see the first few weeks after surgery?

If you are still concerned, ask your surgeon if you can see several patients during the first few weeks of recovery. Most will need sutures removed and will be happy to speak with you.

Blood and bleeding

Blood is composed of many cells, antibodies, hormones, and other essential components. Of primary importance is the oxygen-carrying capacity of red blood cells. Bright red blood cells have plenty of oxygen; those blue veins you see in your arms and hands are filled with spent blood cells that are returning to your lungs for more oxygen. This red blood cell chain is a food cart of sorts that assures your body receives critically important chemical nutrition. Without adequate blood flow, the wounded tissue cannot be fed and healed.

We must have a good blood supply to perform surgery safely, and, if possible, the operation should not jeopardize the circulation of the surgical site. In the fatal liposuction cases that have occurred, the patient's circulation had been dramatically compromised; fluid loss leads to shock and possible death.

Obviously, some degree of bleeding will occur when an artery, vein, or capillary is severed. Luckily, the average healthy person has natural protective mechanisms to intervene and halt bleeding: Blood vessels narrow, and the blood clots.

Bruising is a natural part of healing

Some people get through surgery without much bruising. I've seen a number of patients who could be described as virtually bruise-free two days after surgery. They are the rare exceptions, however. Yes, any number of surgery techniques and better medications are reducing the overall amount of general bruising some people experience. However, even in the best hands, you'll likely have some blue or purple, even brown, blotching. These uneven blotches are simple bruising, caused by local bleeding or blood pooling below the skin.

Bruising seems to be more common after general anesthesia than local anesthesia. One reason may be because medications such as epinephrine that narrow blood vessels can be given with the local anesthetic to lessen bleeding. General anesthetic seems to widen blood vessels, although this delivery system is continually being refined and great strides are taking place in the field of general anesthesia. Most bruising gradually diminishes within two to three weeks of surgery, but there is variation. Some bruising seems to be completely gone after a week. Rarely do major areas of bruising continue much after four or five weeks after surgery.

Fortunately, in most cases there are ways to minimize the degree of bleeding and bruising. Apart from medicines used at the time of the operation to help minimize blood flow, individual vessel ligation or cautery also helps. This is rare in most cosmetic procedures, however.

It's worth repeating: Because aspirin is a blood thinner, you should avoid taking it after surgery,

Bright Idea
Carefully applied pressure dressings, careful surgery, and delicate suturing may minimize the amount of bruising. Drink plenty of water postoperatively to assure the healthy flow of fluids. Your circulation essentially whisks away the deposits of old blood that creates the blue, brown, and purple shades.

which will help minimize bruising. Your surgeon will give you medication to control any postoperative pain. Since a few other drugs can also impair the function of platelets that are necessary for blood clotting, it's wise to show all of your prescriptions to your surgeon. Determine which ones must be avoided and for how long before your elective operation.

Blood transfusions

Most adults have about five quarts of whole blood in their body. Loss of a pint can be tolerated easily and the body will simply manufacture new red blood cells for replacement. Even if the procedure is minor, drink plenty of water several days before your surgery. And, depending on when your surgeon dictates no more liquids (usually midnight before the day of your surgery), make sure your last drink is water. Make it a generous one. Depending on scheduling, your operation may be delayed because of someone else's emergency. Use the extra day or two to hydrate yourself!

Since one pint of blood is the amount donated on an elective basis in blood banks, you may wish to explore stocking your own supply prior to surgery. When the chance of blood loss is significantly greater than one pint—typically about a quart or slightly more—blood transfusions are a possibility. This extra precaution is often done for liposuction treatments, especially if your fat removal might exceed the norm. Donating your own blood for storage before surgery eliminates any possibility of contracting AIDS or hepatitis through a transfusion.

Your role in recovery

It's amazing how many patients destroy or jeopardize their recovery by doing stupid things. One young woman I know had a tummy tuck and thigh liposuction on a Monday. She stayed in a hospital out of town and, upon being discharged, she was told to rest before returning to the surgeon's office in several days for her follow-up visit. Instead, she took a cab to the airport, lifting her own luggage as she raced to catch an airplane. She ripped her sutures immediately and began to bleed profusely. Within an hour she was back in the hospital—in the emergency room!

As cases like this show, it's important to remember that *you* are largely responsible for your own recovery. All the care that the surgeon takes during the surgery won't mean a thing unless you take proper care of your healing afterward.

Age counts

Unofficially...
For an older patient with no systemic problem (such as diabetes), the healing success rate is as good as the norm.

Older patients often give cosmetic surgery the postoperative respect it deserves. Much anecdotal information (as well as clinical studies) suggests that older patients take longer to heal than younger patients. However, in cosmetic surgery, some older patients show more sense than their younger counterparts! They value how their bodies respond, take nothing for granted, and usually appreciate, despite their years, that the doctor actually may know what's best when assigning protocol. Older patients, especially women, can be more conservative and able to evaluate healing risks better. Many are quick to spot questionable responses to medicine and healing. However, because skin becomes thinner as we age, older patients must take greater care to avoid putting stress on the sutures.

Nutrition and following a healthy diet

I recall reading a wonderful short story by a young writer who was languishing in Africa. The area had been suffering from a drought for years and the land was unable to sustain much vegetation, much less animal life. He had a small cut on his leg, which eventually festered. The wound simply would not heal and remained open. A doctor offered a simple explanation. In order for the man's wound to close, he needed a diet with some protein. Without protein, the body cannot heal itself. "Oh" was the writer's next sentence. (Oh, indeed!)

Cellular membranes, which are involved in inflammation and other phases of wound healing, require essential unsaturated fatty acids. Fat is also a component of cell membranes. Although not as widely studied as other dietary deficiencies, fatty acid deficiencies have been shown to cause delayed wound healing in man and in animals.

Some of the vitamins and minerals that promote healing include:

- *Vitamin A.* A deficiency in vitamin A can alter healthy collagen production and contribute to infection.

- *Vitamin B.* A deficiency of vitamin B (riboflavin, pyridoxine, thiamin) can limit collagen production.

- *Vitamin K.* A vitamin K deficiency may reduce the ability of the blood to clot.

- *Iron.* Low iron levels may reduce the transporting of oxygen.

- *Copper.* A deficiency in copper may compromise collagen formation.

- *Zinc.* Low zinc levels may inhibit epithelialization and fibroblast proliferation.

Don't load up on vitamins without your surgeon's permission. And obviously, your recuperation is no time to diet, skimp on nutrients, and hasten weight loss.

Be vigilant about infection

For all types of surgery, wound infection is a potential risk. Bacteria are invisible and, despite the appearance of pristine conditions and a sterile environment, they do find their way into an open wound. In the majority of cases, the body's own defense mechanisms (cellular and biochemical) destroy bacteria to prevent them from multiplying into infections.

Oddly enough, for standard clean operations, preoperative antibiotics do not decrease the chances of infection. In fact, such nonspecific antibiotic administration can lower certain immune responses and actually increase the likelihood of infections by bacteria that are difficult to treat and resistant to the common medications.

Fortunately, wound infections are rare. If they do occur, they usually respond promptly to surgical drainage (wound opening) and judicious medications.

Sterile dressings

In practically all elective cosmetic surgery, immediately at the end of each procedure, sterile dressings are placed on the wound. Invariably, this will be done while you're still under anesthesia and lying on the operating table. Dressings can differ greatly, with the most popular types including:

- A small adhesive bandage that is easily removed
- A soft piece of tape that leaves no adhesive when removed
- Elaborate gauze wrappings
- Elastic bandages

If the dressing is to be left intact, patients must keep the dressings dry and reasonably clean. If the dressing is to be removed or changed, be sure you receive careful instructions on how to do so. Know exactly which type of new dressing should be applied, and where and how it should be done.

Postoperative medications

Almost every patient is given some postoperative pain medication, except in the case of very minor surgery. Very rarely are antibiotics prescribed. Most elective operations do not require an antibiotic because the wounds are clean. The surgical environment is sterile and often the procedure is called "clean surgery."

Elevation and sutures

All patients should expect some normal swelling after surgery. Keeping certain areas and limbs elevated will minimize excessive swelling.

In general, the surgical site should be elevated for two or three days after surgery. This means that if the surgery is on the face, you should sleep with your head elevated, comfortably propped with pillows.

Almost all wounds are sutured and, in cosmetic surgery, most sutures have to be removed. There are many types of removable sutures and most are made of a synthetic substance that causes very little, if any, scarring. Most come in basic black, which can be alarming to see if you're unprepared. Sutures can also be made of metal and resemble staples. These rarely leave marks if used properly and are easy to remove; they essentially slide out.

Dissolving sutures are used most often for surgery on areas of the body such as the breast or abdomen. They are sometimes used below the skin inside the mouth. These sutures dissolve naturally over time and tend to leave slightly more scarring than sutures that must be removed.

Sutures can stay in place from several days to a few weeks. In the eyelids, most sutures are removed within four to five days, but for brow lifts and several other procedures sutures will remain in place longer. The correct time for suture removal is dictated by three variables:

1. Your healing ability

2. Wound tension created by the suture

3. Your surgeon's recommendation

You will be given an appointment to return to the office for removal of the sutures, usually five to seven days after surgery. Never hesitate to have a nurse remove stitches. It is painless and they are much better at it than most surgeons. Trust them!

Fastidiously follow protocol

Be sure to discuss with your surgeon any activities that you should avoid during the recovery period. If you're in doubt, ask.

Usually activities that do not produce any discomfort are not harmful. Nature's protective mechanisms produce pain to tell us when we are being too active after surgery. However, specific restrictions, such as sweating while your sutures are still in and other protocols, must be discussed with your doctor. Protocol will vary greatly with each patient and type of operation.

Postsurgery follow-up

After surgery, most patients see their doctor on more than one occasion for follow-up visits. However, very minor operations may require only

Watch Out!
Normal wound healing under most circumstances takes about six weeks. During this period, stay away from the gym! Strenuous activity should be avoided. You must repair yourself inside and out.

one follow-up visit after five to seven days for suture removal. At that time, long-term precautions, such as avoiding the sun and make-up application, can be discussed. Keep a list of questions and discuss them with your doctor during the visit.

If the operation has been more extensive, more follow-up visits will be necessary, perhaps after six weeks when primary healing can be assessed.

You may be asked to return a number of months or even a year after surgery, when all postoperative changes have taken place. At that time, have your final results photographed and take a peek at your preoperative photos—you may not believe the difference!

If there are complications, you may need to see your doctor for more frequent follow-up visits. You and the surgeon can work together to promote healing and a satisfactory final outcome.

After surgery, you should always feel free to contact the surgeon or a member of the medical team at any time. Know the office phone number and the number of the surgeon or on-call physician. Make sure your family or contact person has the number readily available; write it down in a permanent place. Carry it with you at all times. Even weeks, months, or years after surgery patients should not hesitate to discuss any questions that might arise.

Just the facts

- Wound healing is best managed by following your doctor's protocol carefully.
- Some swelling and bruising of the surgical site are normal and should be expected.
- Give scars up to a year before you assess the final healing results.

- You can make your recovery go more smoothly by following a healthy diet, keeping the wound clean, and being careful not to disturb the sutures.

- Keep all follow-up visits scheduled by your surgeon.

GET THE SCOOP ON...
You're back in charge! ▪ Exploring aftercare
options ▪ Your postoperative tool kit ▪ Making
good use of your recovery time ▪ In a funk:
dealing with postsurgery blues and stress ▪
Following up with your doctor

Managing Postoperative Discomfort

Each of us heals and feels differently following surgery. In this chapter I'll give you some great coping techniques to manage your recovery. The more you can do to prepare yourself prior to your surgery, the better your healing process and your satisfaction with the results will be.

Earlier on in your search, you did a lot of sleuthing and checking to make sure your aesthetic needs would be addressed by the best surgeon and best recommended methodology. After that take-charge period, most patients—due to stress, very busy and demanding lives, and general fatigue—happily surrender the morning of their surgery. You've chosen an expert, capable surgeon to take over. You're ready. But as you nervously sign a number of documents that give you the willies when you think about the ramifications of something going wrong, you realize you're no longer in control.

Don't fret; those are actually healthy and perfectly normal thoughts. Other patients feel nothing but exhilaration and pride. The range of reactions and mood swings varies considerably by patient, by procedure, and by other variables too. However, here's the good news: You're now back in charge!

You'll need to monitor your aftercare fastidiously; this chapter's inside tips help make the interim healing period work in your favor. You'll also learn how to rest comfortably until you can resume your regular sleeping position, how to wisely maximize your follow-up visits, and how simple exercise following surgery can put you ahead of the game. And since you're back in charge, remember: It's your responsibility, and yours alone, to follow your doctor's protocol with great discipline. So, if you're feeling punk after surgery and if you don't want to feel worse and slip into a nasty depression, this chapter is for you.

Making the most of aftercare

As you've learned, the wisest thing you can do for yourself is to prepare *before* surgery for your return. But there is also a growing trend for many patients to seek refuge in a retreat—sometimes known as a hideaway—to get the best aftercare possible. Celebrities often check in under assumed names and only a few staff members, if any, are aware of their presence. Recuperating at a recovery retreat is a trend that's destined to increase. In the future, it's likely that a number of doctors will develop their own on-site hideaways.

Recovery at retreats

There are several cosmetic surgery hideaways listed in Appendix B. To appreciate the services these places offer, let's take a closer look at one of the best: *Le Palais Chantique,* Los Angeles' premier recovery retreat. The discrete organization caters to both men and women who simply want to vanish after surgery but who want to have the best postoperative care. Located on the sixth floor of the Beverly Prescott Hotel, the facility features a discreet pickup and delivery service with both a chauffeur and nurse who make the trip from the hospital safe and comfortable. You are speedily transported to the retreat's private entrance and personal elevator. There are about a dozen rooms tucked quietly away and each is beautifully designed with all top amenities and round-the-clock nursing care. Fees range around $400 per night; there are varied plans and packages available. Meals are beautifully prepared and the correct amount of body movement and mild exercise are monitored by experts. Your privacy is guarded and no other patient sees you coming and going.

Some doctors are beginning to offer postoperative care at their own hideaway retreats. One of the better state-of-the-art retreats is owned and operated by Dr. Robert N. Cooper in Florida. Following surgery, Dr. Cooper sees each patient twice a day at the retreat. He also visits New York City once a month to consult with interested prospects. As with all surgical services, you must be careful to study the credentials and expertise of all staff and not be swayed by issues that have little to do with managing risk and aftercare.

Recovery at home

Before surgery, your bedroom should be equipped and ready for your arrival. Chapter 4 specifies some of the things to do beforehand. Barbara Rhea is an expert registered nurse whose specialty is cosmetic surgery recovery. She has worked with many celebrities, often travels the country to provide expert

Unofficially...
Since three areas—southern California, Florida, and metropolitan New York—are key areas for having cosmetic surgery, you're more likely to find a greater number of aftercare services in these areas. But Nashville, Chicago, and Atlanta also have thriving aftercare markets that cater to cosmetic surgery recovery.

postoperative care, and is in great demand by top surgeons. Here's what Nurse Rhea recommends as important, must-have items; keep them within easy access. You'll need:

- A copy of your doctor's protocol and any prescriptions for medicines you'll need after surgery
- Tylenol, Benadryl, and stool softener medicine, as needed
- Latex gloves and baby lima beans (Intrigued? Keep reading!)
- A disposable cooler for holding small, loose cubes of ice, cool drinks such as water or juice, and a soft-food diet such as yogurt
- Clean, soft, thin cloths or baby washcloths
- Bendable straws for easy sipping of liquids
- Witch hazel or white vinegar
- Kerlix (or cotton only) gauze and soft, medical adhesive tape for dressing the surgical site
- Cotton swabs
- Two or three large, clean towels

Here's what to do with this postoperative tool kit.

First, have any prescriptions filled before your surgery or make sure your pharmacy can deliver the prescription. If the latter, have someone at home with you to receive the delivery should you be sleeping. Keep a copy of your doctor's protocol by your bedside for any aftercare person to refer to.

Before going into the hospital, take several latex gloves—perhaps half a dozen or so—and fill them halfway with baby lima beans. Don't plump the contents, but pat the gloves flat and then place them in the freezer. These make excellent cold compresses and can be refrozen. (A small bag of frozen peas also makes a good cold compress.) Always use a moist barrier cloth—soft, clean, and thin—between the cold compress and your skin. To each moist cloth, if you like, add a few drops of witch hazel or white vinegar for a refreshing feel.

Place one large towel over your pillow case or the resting area close to the surgical site. This will help keep your bedding clean as the wound heals itself. Keep a pair of socks handy; your feet will invariably get cold. An extra blanket is a good backup, too. Keep your window open to eliminate stuffiness.

Soft foods such as rice pudding and mashed potatoes will help your digestive system get back on track. Eating yogurt, according to Nurse Rhea, is a great way to restore those digestive stomach enzymes which may have been eliminated or diminished by the anesthetic. Flexible straws make drinking liquids easier; you'll be surprised how hard it may be to simply lift your head. Many patients experience constipation following cosmetic surgery. In these instances, a mild stool softener may help ease any discomfort. Drinking a reasonable amount of water will also help—it keeps the lower tract from drying up.

Getting back to a comfortable sleeping routine

Although the body wants to recover and values the healing ability of sound sleep, some patients find it difficult to resume their normal sleeping pattern. If you have trouble sleeping, taking a simple antihistamine such as Benadryl may be all you need to nod off (but check with your doctor before taking it or any medication that hasn't been prescribed). Other simple remedies such as drinking chamomile tea or warm milk may also help, as can some of the

Timesaver
Follow the "20-20" cold-compress formula for success: Apply a cold compress to the wound for 20 minutes, then leave it off for 20 minutes. Repeat this as often as possible for the first 24 to 48 hours to keep swelling and bruising to a minimum.

following tips. However, if insomnia remains a problem, your doctor may recommend a mild sedative for the short term.

Depending on the area in which you had surgery, you may not be able to sleep in your usual position for the first week or so following surgery. Keeping the head elevated significantly reduces swelling and postoperative bruising that attend any face surgery. You may think this is an impossible accommodation for your body to make at this time, but expect to be surprised. Sleeping upright with plenty of pillows to brace you provides a comforting, cradlelike sensation as your circulation runs its course to promote healing. Depending on your surgery, your doctor's protocol is designed to place your body in the best resting position to keep swelling to a minimum.

Some people report an extreme restlessness the first night. Their limbs, mostly the legs and thighs, may ache very mildly. In most cases, stretching your legs helps—sit upright at the edge of your bed and let your ankles and toes dangle. In other cases, taking a short, slow stroll on the arm of a nurse will cause this "antsy" feeling to pass. Even if you get up three or four times, you'll find that you'll be able to return to sleep. If you notice that your breathing is rapid and short while you're in bed, there may be an emotional or stress-related trigger. You should take two or three deep breaths and exhale slowly. Here are several other tips for inducing sleep:

- Limit your intake of caffeine before bed. Avoid drinks such as coffee, tea, or cola.

- Avoid alcohol during your recovery period. It may induce a drowsy feeling, but after a short time you may be wide awake again.

- Keep the room at a comfortable temperature and leave a window open to keep air circulating.

Don't skimp now: get a pro

It is absolutely essential that you have a reliable, qualified aftercare aide to manage your adjustment if your surgery has been major. If you've had a face lift, tummy tuck, or other significant procedure, you must have a registered nurse to look after you for the first 24 hours.

If you're in a hospital, the regular staff will be able to vigilantly attend to your needs. If you are being sent home following your surgery, you must have someone with RN credentials to follow your progress if your surgeon advises you to do so. You cannot manage this aspect of your recovery by yourself. Here are four reasons why:

1. Your final healing and scars may be compromised.

2. You will be too drowsy or weak to follow medical protocol.

3. Recovery means rest and restricted movement; you can't rest *and* attend to postoperative care.

4. You may overlook the development of a hematoma or other potential problem.

To arrange for a postoperative aftercare nurse, ask your surgeon for a recommendation or check with your local hospital or hospital referral service.

The average cost for a top registered nurse to see you through the first night and well into the next morning ranges from $300 to $500. Unbelievably, this is where some patients begin to cut corners and place themselves at risk. Don't do it!

The following three real-life cases of patients ignoring doctor protocol illustrate the importance of proper aftercare:

Watch Out!
Be careful! There are a number of home-care attendants who lack medical training and are *not* qualified to treat or recognize developing problems. Don't relegate your initial 24-hour postoperative watch to a home-care attendant who is not a qualified registered nurse.

- A well-intentioned neighbor mistook a friend's clear lip gloss for prescription eye ointment. The neighbor applied the lip gloss to her friend's eyelids, and one of her swollen lids became infected.

- After having breast implants, a Dallas art director told her surgeon she was heading home where a registered nurse awaited her. Instead, she and a girlfriend went shopping and then celebrated her new look with margaritas. The former patient, dehydrated by the alcohol and still weak from the surgery, wound up fainting, cutting her eye and forehead in the fall.

- Following minor chin liposuction, a marketing executive jumped into his club's sauna "just to break a sweat" before heading home. Still foggy from the local anesthetic, he used a loofah to abrade his five o'clock shadow and popped two sutures.

Recovery is a collaborative effort. Following your doctor's protocol and using common sense should minimize any problems.

Making yourself comfortable

The type of surgery you have will determine how you can lull away the recovery hours. For example, with breast implants, a nose job, or a face lift, you'll want to rest only the first day or so. By the second or third day, you might want to watch a little TV as you nap. More serious surgery—tummy tucks and significant liposuction—will require your doing very little for several days. And you won't want to do much more than just sleep and eat a little. Eye or nose jobs, even face lifts, will preclude you from wearing contact lenses or even eyeglasses. Simple reading may be out of the question for many patients.

Before undergoing surgery, give some thought to some special treats that will lift your spirits or keep you busy for short periods. Obviously explore options that easily fit into your doctor's protocol, but make a specific list of four or five things that make you feel good—perhaps a favorite brand of ice cream, a new music CD, or some brightly colored pillows to prop you up in bed.

Make specific plans to carry you through your recovery. If you love flowers, treat yourself to a new bouquet every day. Aromatherapy can also help elevate your mood. Schedule some short visits with close friends who can drop in and offer support and amusing distraction.

It's amazing how creative some patients are in making this recovery time a productive, healthful period. One Arizona accountant—who had a neck lift as well as a lower lid eye job—used his 10-day recovery time to study Italian music. He always had an interest in it and took his superficial knowledge to an almost scholarly level within two weeks. He ordered composer biographies on audio tapes and bought rare Maria Callas recordings of Puccini and Verde. A 39-year-old Seattle food importer finally learned biofeedback, the relaxation technique her therapist had recommended four years prior. She recalls, "I never had the time. And then, wham! I had two weeks of napping and rest." She jokes that her life has changed remarkably, but she'll never know if it was the surgery or the biofeedback.

Beating the postsurgery blues

Depression is a part of recovery for many patients. Even the most blithe spirit can be caught off guard by some odd funk that pops up without any warning. Of course, you may breeze through this period

Bright Idea
If you like to read but know you won't be able to during the recovery period, buy a book on audio cassette before the surgery so you can listen to it as you recuperate. Check your local bookstore for a wide variety of interesting books available on audio cassettes.

without one down moment. But, rather than having it strike without warning, if you have some safety nets in place prior to the negative mood swing, you'll be able to cope better.

There are many reasons why cosmetic surgery patients may feel blue. Here are five common contributors:

1. Great anticipation and eventual stress levels often create a rebound effect.

2. Medications, anesthetic, and body trauma can make you feel out of sorts.

3. Limited exercise during recovery contributes to a sense of feeling powerless and blue.

4. You may be unprepared for how you'll look immediately following surgery.

5. Many patients harbor a hidden fear of disfigurement following surgery.

Usually this mild depression vanishes within a day or so at most; for many it passes in an afternoon or a few hours. Remember, this depression is *endogenous*, meaning the cause is likely to be physiological and traceable to some aspect of your surgery. It should not be confused with *exogenous* depression, which is traceable to a significant event such as a death of a loved one, loss of a job, or a personally troubling situation such as financial woes.

Let's talk about some of the things you can do to create a better sense of well-being and eliminate your fleeting blue funk.

Relaxation techniques

As ironic as it may seem, you may need to learn how to relax. Here's a technique that helps you do just that. Lie flat, if possible, keeping your body loose and your legs about hip-width apart. Your arms should be relaxed, palms upward. Close your eyes and keep your mouth slightly open Flatten your shoulder blades comfortably, avoiding the natural hunch we all fall into when we are tense. Let your body simply flow. Imagine healthy, bright energy, a clear, sky-blue healing source that enters through the top of your body and paces itself throughout all your limbs and downward through your tummy. As the energy pours through your body, it moves through tension and pain, gently circulating in massaging circles to cleanse your spirit. Think of this energy as a cleansing flow that removes all pain, distress, and tension. Slowly curl your toes downward and toward yourself. As you do this, your body begins to feel rested, cleansed, and lighter.

Simple breathing techniques also help. Relax and inhale very slowly through your nose. Keep your eyes closed and listen to the deep breathing process. Let your lungs fill deeply, hold for a brief moment, and then very slowly exhale through your mouth. Release the breath slowly and evenly. Repeat this deep breathing three times, feeling yourself become more relaxed.

Managing stress

In the early phases of any recovery, there's one simple rule: If you feel pain, stop what you're doing. The same can be said for whatever causes mental stress. And this is truly an area you can manage. For example, if the office is apt to bug you at home and make you worry about an unhappy client, don't take the calls.

Until your recovery is well underway, you can choose who and what is permitted to intrude on your recovery. Most stress during this period is avoidable. Remember: You're in control! So, react

Bright Idea
If you're feeling stressed by being away from the office, have an answering machine in another room to take all incoming phone messages. Turn down the volume. Keep away from unnecessary incoming messages until you feel up to dealing with work.

only to those situations that you must; save your energy for combating what is unavoidable. Put problems out of your mind. The same goes for difficult circumstances and demanding people.

Understand that stress weakens both your recovery and overall performance. In the section on exercise, later in this chapter, you'll learn how simple exercise can be one of life's best stress relievers.

Making the most of follow-up visits

You're now ready to see your doctor following the surgery. You know what you want to say. But will your surgeon really hear you? Clearly, if you've had the speediest recovery possible and are so pleased with your results, the gist of this message will get conveyed. But what if you have a few concerns?

In many ways, patients can help their cause by observing a few smart details during their follow-up visits. There are several "no-no's," too. I talked to many doctors as well as to their office managers, nurses, and other medical staff to see how you can get the treatment you need and deserve. Here's what the pros suggest:

- *Remember that it's an office of professionals, not underlings.* Treat the receptionist and support staff with respect. Know their names and don't lose your cool when trying to explain your concern.

- *Understand that you are one of many people the doctor serves.* Appointments may back up if there is an emergency or the staff is short that day. Be patient and you'll find most people will work harder for you.

- *Be prepared.* Yes, your surgery cost a lot but that doesn't buy unlimited access to meandering discussions and woe-is-me consultations. Your physician's time is limited. The more prepared you are, the better the care can be tailored to your situation. If there is a symptom that appears out of the norm, be able to describe the symptom and when and how it manifests itself.

■ *Bring notes.* Write down any questions you have; it's easier to cover them at once rather than following up with several phone calls. Don't ramble and bring up issues that are not relevant to the situation you are addressing.

Here are the most common gaffs that work against you:

■ *Ignoring instructions.* Deciding not to comply with your surgeon's recommendation strains the doctor-patient relationship. By ignoring protocol, you're essentially saying, "I don't agree," "I know better," "I don't trust you," or "I don't care." If you have questions about a doctor's recommendation, discuss the issues you have when the protocol is first proposed. Ignoring the doctor marks you as a difficult and potentially dangerous patient.

■ *Showing up late for the visit.* Yes, we all know that many doctors are behind schedule and unable to see patients at the appointed time. It's an unfortunate fact of life in many offices. Now is not the time to overhaul the system. If you want to be treated well, you must be prompt.

■ *Arguing and becoming adversarial.* Knowing how to cope with your situation and using effective people skills are key to your getting the results you expected. Threatening a doctor, screaming, or becoming antagonistic will make it difficult, if not impossible, to achieve your goal. Much of the medical field has a higher-than-average

Unofficially...
Doctors and staff alike say that a simple handwritten thank-you note or small bouquet of flowers are never expected. But when a small token of appreciation does arrive, it's amazing how well the patient who sent it is treated.

burnout factor. Contributing to the stress level by hassling the staff or badgering your doctor only works against you.

■ *Talking negatively about results.* It's a common mistake for patients to suddenly notice some slight irregularities as they go through the recovery period. But remember, many of the things you'll begin to notice may already have been there prior to surgery. I remember a friend feeling her nose became crooked after she had her brow lift. The fact is, it was always slightly crooked (thankfully, she was able to locate a presurgery photograph to confirm this fact and to calm her misplaced anxiety). It's important to discuss these concerns with your doctor and his staff—it's part of your surgical care and the fee you paid.

If you see something that isn't quite even, don't panic. Swelling doesn't subside equally and on any predictable schedule. The left side of your body might outpace the right side. You must be able to weather this period, which can take up to a year. Accept your surgeon's assurances and use his or her expectations to measure your results. And never compare your recovery to that of someone else who had the same surgery. There is no equitable way to make this comparison.

■ *Insisting your surgeon handle suture removal.* Sutures, staples, and screws slide out in a most amazing fashion, lubricated in part by the soft inside of the healing body. There is no pain or stinging. It's worth repeating: If a nurse is available to remove your sutures and your doctor suggests it, go with the nurse over the doctor any day! It's likely the nurse has much more experience in suture removal. I believe most do a better job.

▪ *Requesting minisurgical revisions.* Please resist any temptation to have your surgeon redo any incision for at least nine months or longer. Even the reddest raised scar has a remarkable ability to flatten out and fade to pale. In most cases, the scar will become quite thin, almost as narrow as silk thread. Any reputable surgeon will include some postoperative revision if you feel it will help (ask before surgery!). If there is an aspect to your surgery that you find bothersome, talk to your doctor and see what revision can be attempted to allay your concern. (Review Chapter 15 so that you can better appreciate how many scars are better left to heal on their own.)

Taking care of yourself

Many patients develop an unusual resolve following cosmetic surgery. The number of patients who adopt an improved diet and develop an overall healthier lifestyle continues to grow each year. There are several reasons. Because surgery is expensive, prospects wish to protect their investment. They truly understand the value of sun block and appreciate how even tropical shade can damage the skin. Here's what has worked in recent years to help many people enjoy a better lifestyle after cosmetic surgery.

Sleep and a healthy diet

As we're all aware, there is a strong correlation between getting enough rest and looking your best. Simple catnaps in the office have great restorative

Watch Out!
Americans, according to recent studies, are a sleep-deprived nation. Most healthy adults could do with an extra one to two hours of sleep each night!

benefits. You need not fall asleep. Simply find a comfortable place to put your feet up and close your eyes. Doing this each day for 20 minutes can carry you through the afternoon with greater verve.

Following surgery, eating a healthier diet becomes easier for many prospects. They feel greater resolve and find their improved appearance is the best motivation for losing extra weight. Whenever you diet and start to lose weight, it's wise to give yourself an extra hour of sleep each night. Your body simply needs it to bounce back with enough energy to propel you through the next day. Without enough sleep during weight loss, you may experience negative mood swings and food cravings that can catch you off guard and sabotage your efforts.

Getting enough exercise

Regular exercise can slow several key aspects in aging—such as muscle loss and diminishing bone mass—and a simple program can help you feel much younger than your years. There are many ways to stay fit and enough spas and gyms to help jump-start any novice's first exercise program.

The obvious and easiest option for most people is a walking workout. Start with a 10-minute walk and then add a few minutes each week. How far and how fast you go depend on establishing and maintaining weekly realistic goals. To boost your health and reduce your risk of contracting numerous chronic diseases, your final goal should be to exercise close to half an hour a day, five or six times a week. And some good news: You can break this amount into several shorter bouts and still reap the same benefits!

Here are five ways to get the most from your walking workout:

1. Take quicker, not longer, steps.

2. Bend your arms and let your hands swing in an arc from your waist upward to your chest.

3. Walk tall by stretching your spine and looking forward; never slouch.

4. Land on your heel, roll forward to and then push off with your toes.

5. Make the route scenic and add a slope or gentle hill for more of a workout. Don't carry ankle or wrist weights, because they can do more harm than good if you don't know how to move your body correctly while using them.

Make sure that you have comfortable walking gear. Look for a pair of athletic shoes designed just for walking. When you shop, bring along the walking socks you'll use and make sure there's a thumb-width distance between the tip of your toes and the shoe's end. The heel should be snug—not tight—and there should be enough light wiggle room for the rest of the foot.

If you are keen on getting in shape but have tried many times in the past, before you begin a program, try to see if you can figure out why your plans end up being scrubbed. Fitness expert Timothy Callaghan says there are four variables that factor into a person's success with exercise. Can you spot which are the two most important? You may be fooled:

■ Patience

■ Motivation

■ Pacing

■ Commitment

Most people would say that motivation is the most important of these factors. If you lose your resolve, how can you continue? Experts say that motivation comes and goes like the monthly lunar pattern. Some days you are wildly motivated. You don't need to get pushed in the direction of the gym. But this same motivation changes over time. Commitment, however, is truly different. Commitment is the real driving force. And when it is coupled with patience, these two skills help you form a habit that you can keep up when motivation lags on certain days. In fact, patience and commitment also deliver the third most important factor: pacing. Pacing, how you get through your day or any other plan, is a result of your personal commitment and ability to use patience to achieve your goal.

No doubt, having successfully completed the entire process of cosmetic surgery, you're already an expert at pacing—and well on your way to a healthy, happy recovery.

Just the facts

- A healthy, smart recovery is something that you can create.
- Depression following cosmetic surgery is common; have a game plan to combat the blues.
- Turn the recovery period into a productive period.
- Act responsibly with protocol; be a compliant patient.
- Getting plenty of sleep, eating a healthy diet, and getting enough exercise are the best ways to stay healthy and enjoy better postoperative results.

Appendices

PART VII

Glossary

abdominal etching   A UAL technique in which a surgeon creates a muscular, rippled appearance on the stomach.

acetone   A liquid solvent often used before cosmetic surgery to remove natural oily deposits on the skin.

adjunct procedure   A secondary, usually less demanding surgical operation performed at the same time as the primary operation; chin liposuction is often an adjunct to a face lift.

AHA (alpha-hydroxy acid)   An exfoliant, often derived from fruit, milk, or other natural sources, that speeds up the shedding of superficial skin cells, leaving the complexion with a smoother, fresher appearance. Medical remedies use an AHA concentration of 30 to 70 percent; beauty counter products average 10 percent or less.

alar nasal cartilage   The wing-shaped cartilage that makes up the tip of the nose.

anesthesia   Loss of sensation in the body induced by administration of a drug. Types of anesthetics generally used in plastic surgery procedures include *local, local with sedation,* and *general* (see separate listings).

antiseptic   A topical substance that prevents or slows the growth of organisms that cause infection; a disinfectant.

aspiration   The surgical removal of a liquid from the body by sucking the fluid through a needle.

asymmetric   Lacking anatomical proportion or balance; uneven.

bacterial infection   Disease-producing contamination caused by germs.

Betadine   An antiseptic used to kill bacteria in the surgical site; often applied to the scalp, for example, prior to a brow lift or face lift.

biomembrane tape   A bandage impregnated with proprietary drugs used to retain moisture, reduce pain, and speed healing.

Botox   A trade name for an injectable substance that paralyzes the muscles that create forehead creases, wrinkles, or even neck muscles that cause the appearance of aging.

breast implant   A silicone rubber shell (today filled with saline solution for cosmetic surgeries only) used to enlarge the breast.

breast lift (mastopexy)   The surgical removal of sagging skin and tissue of the breast to modify the pendulous appearance, possibly correcting any attending chronic discomfort.

breast reduction (mammoplasty) A surgical procedure performed to reduce the size of the breast.

brow lift The surgical repositioning and reshaping of the eyebrow and/or forehead. See *coronal lift*.

cannula A small probing tube used during liposuction to remove fat by suction.

certification A statement by a medical board that a surgeon is qualified to perform an operation in that board's specialty. The term also applies to surgical facilities that have met certain health standards established by government agencies.

charring Scorching or burning of the skin caused by older laser techniques.

chemical peel (chemosurgery) Removal of unwanted skin layers by means of chemicals, to promote the regrowth of fresh, less wrinkled or marred new skin.

chin lift Generally the removal of fat (and, in some cases, excess skin) that detracts from jaw line definition.

collagen The major protein of connective tissue that helps make up the foundation of skin and other tissues. When extracted from animal skin, it is used as an injectable filler to plump depressed areas or augment deficient areas of the skin.

conjunctiva The lining of the eyelids and eye.

connective tissue Ligaments, tendons, or muscle sheaths.

coronal lift   A surgical procedure done above the forehead to remove excess skin, lift the brow, and thereby diminish or eliminate wrinkles and frown lines.

cosmetic surgery   An elective operation done solely to improve one's appearance.

crow's feet   Wrinkles at the outside corners of the eyes; often a secondary procedure to a face lift or blepharoplasty is required to specifically treat these wrinkles.

dermabrasion   An operation to remove the outer layers of the skin by abrasion so that the new skin growth will improve imperfections such as wrinkles or acne scars.

dermatolipectomy   Surgical removal of excess skin and fat.

dermatologist   A physician who specializes in the treatment of skin disorders.

ectropion   An abnormal turning out of an eyelid causing an appearance like that of a bloodhound or basset hound; an undesirable complication that can occur after lower lid eye surgery if too much skin is removed.

Endermologie   A nonsurgical methodology involving a series of treatments that reduce (through heat and mechanical rolling devices) the appearance of fat that often accumulates in thighs, upper arms, and other areas.

endoscope   A microscopic optical instrument (miniature video camera in a small tube hooked up to a monitor screen) which can be inserted through a small incision during surgery, permitting the surgeon to see and perform critical operation steps such as suturing, or locating and placing implants. An endoscope is used in many cosmetic procedures—forehead lifts, breast implants, face lifts, tummy tucks, among others—and typically results in less postoperative swelling, bruising, and discomfort.

endoscopic facioplasty   A face lift that is done using endoscopy.

endoscopic lift   Any surgical lift that is done using endoscopy.

epinephrine   Same as adrenaline, used chiefly to control bleeding and to prolong the effect of local anesthetics. It works by constricting the blood vessels.

excision   The surgical removal of tissue, usually by cutting.

exfoliation   The removal of upper skin in thin layers; chemicals, Retin-A, and facial granular scrubs are exfoliating products.

eye job (blepharoplasty)   Cosmetic surgery performed on the eyelids, involving the removal of fat and/or skin, usually to reduce signs of aging.

face lift (facioplasty)   A surgical operation that is usually performed on the lower part of the face to remove creases and tighten sagging skin, resulting in a smoother, younger appearance.

face peel   The removal of skin layers from the face, usually by abrasion, chemicals, or laser, so new skin can grow and give a more aesthetic result.

facial implant surgery An operation to insert bone, cartilage, or synthetic material into the face to enhance or balance features such as the lips, chin, cheeks, or nasal labial folds.

facial tic Spasmodic twitching of facial muscles.

fascia Fibrous tissue that is found throughout the body beneath the skin. It encloses muscles and groups of muscles and separates and anchors several tissue layers of the body.

fiber optics The transmission of light through a bundle of glass fibers.

flaccid skin Skin without tone and elasticity.

flap surgery An operation that incises a segment of tissue, skin, fat, or sometimes a muscle or fascia, with the blood vessels and nerves, and moves it to another position. Usually done to improve the outside surface as a cosmetic correction.

Flexzan A proprietary bandage that is soft, pliable, and used following cosmetic surgery to help certain incisions heal.

follicle A small cavity or sac.

forehead lift Surgery that diminishes wrinkles, creases, and signs of aging on the forehead. See *coronal lift*.

frontalis A muscle under the skin of the forehead.

general anesthetic An anesthetic administered to induce sleep; a ventilator is used to assist breathing.

glycolic acid A fruit acid used in chemical peels; available in various concentrations and milder than phenol.

glycolic peel The removal of skin surfaces using a fruit acid; can be performed by dermatologists or other cosmetic doctors.

Gore-Tex A lightweight, durable, synthetic fiber used as a tissue filler or to support tissue.

gynecomastia Excessive breast development in males, which is often a hormonal response; fatty deposits make the breast larger and can produce the appearance of a female breast.

hairband incision A surgical cut in the scalp behind the hairline which goes practically ear to ear. Used in a brow lift, this large incision is being replaced by endoscopic technology.

hematoma A swelling containing blood under the skin; a common postoperative occurrence that often resolves on its own or can be surgically removed.

hemorrhage Heavy, uncontrolled bleeding.

hooding An abnormal appearance of the upper eyelid caused by excessive sagging of the lid skin, often due to aging.

hydroquinone A prescription bleaching agent, commonly used with Retin-A or AHA treatments for management of irregularities in skin pigmentation.

hyperpigmentation An excessive discoloration of the skin.

hypertrophic scar A medical term used to describe a widened or enlarged scar that remains within the boundaries of the initial injury or incision.

implant A surgically placed, permanent insert, usually made of synthetic material, that is used to correct an atanomical deficiency or to restore physical harmony.

keloid   Redundant fibrous tissue that forms at the site of a cut or incision due to an overproduction of collagen.

lagophthalmos   Inability to close one or both eyelids; an undesirable complication to eye-lift surgery, usually traceable to excising too much skin or the result of scarring.

laser   An acronym for Light Amplification by Simulated Emission of Radiation. It concentrates visible light into a very small area and leaves surrounding areas untouched; lasers are used in varied ways, such as to make incisions that barely bleed, to resurface skin, and to remove veins.

laser resurfacing (laser peel)   Surgery that uses a laser beam to eliminate or modify unsightly skin defects.

lidocaine   A local anesthetic.

liposuction   A cosmetic procedure in which excess fat is removed from under skin and tissue by mechanically vacuuming deposits out through a small tube.

local anesthetic   An anesthetic injected to numb the area being treated; often given in conjunction with a mild relaxant taken orally.

local with sedation   Medication administered by vein to induce sleep, followed by an injection of an anesthetic to numb the area being treated.

lymph   A clear fluid that resembles blood plasma, containing white blood cells and no red blood cells.

MAC (monitored-anesthesia control) An adjunct to local anesthetic in which the patient's pulse rate, blood pressure, oxygen saturation, and other critical responses are vigilantly monitored. If necessary, additional sedatives and pain-relieving medications may be dispensed by an intravenous (IV) line, which also provides immediate access if there is an adverse reaction.

marionette lines A term used to describe vertical creases extending from the corners of the mouth to the jaw.

mastoid The bone behind the ear that raises up as a hump and carries much of the stress of lifting sutures in facial cosmetic surgery.

medical board A group of doctors who scrutinize the professional training, education, and credentials of other physicians (such as the ABA, ABMS, ABPS, and ASAPS).

melanin A pigment in the skin that can darken it.

methodology A particular procedure, such as liposuction or resurfacing, used by a cosmetic surgeon.

milia Small whiteheads that may form when the skin is abraded or treated.

minilift A facial rejuvenating procedure in which an incision is made only in the temple area and the skin is redraped. This procedure works best for patients who have no major signs of sagging, deep creases, or wrinkles, which are best corrected by excessive undermining and a full face lift.

nasolabial fold The crease extending from the side of the nostril to the corner of the mouth.

nose job (rhinoplasty)   Cosmetic surgery performed to reshape the contour or size the nose.

Obagi Blue Peel   A facial peel using trichloracetic acid with a blue dye that helps the physician determine the dermal extent of penetration to better control the peeling process.

occlusive gauze   A bandage treated with special medicinal agents to manage bleeding.

ophthalmologist   A physician who specializes in treating eye conditions and eye surgery.

otoplasty   The surgical correction of an ear deformity.

outpatient   A person who receives treatment at a clinic, office, or other facility that treats patients who do not need to stay overnight at a hospital. The term can also be applied to the facility itself (outpatient clinic).

panniculectomy   A surgical procedure that removes large quantities of excess skin and its underlying fat. This procedure can be performed virtually anywhere on the body.

penile enhancement   A surgical procedure to make the penis appear larger.

phenol   A strong chemical used to resurface the skin; the original chemical peel.

plastic surgery   The branch of surgery dealing with the repair or enhancement of malformed, injured, or lost organs or tissues.

platysmal bands   Cords of the neck muscle that extend from the jaw to the collarbone on either side of the neck.

preoperative sedation   Medicine given to relax the patient before the operation.

resection The surgical removal of tissue such as skin and fat.

Retin-A A prescription medication derived from vitamin A, prescribed commonly by a dermatologist for the treatment of acne and used frequently as an exfoliating treatment prior to chemical peels.

robotics Automatic computer-regulated mechanisms that guide and control lasers during surgery.

scalp reduction An operation to reduce areas of baldness by removing hairless scalp and closing the defect created with hair-bearing scalp.

sclerotherapy A technique for treating spider veins by injecting a solution that collapses the vein.

skin resurfacing A surgical procedure that removes upper skin layers to produce new skin. Lasers and peels are two resurfacing methodologies that can diminish acne scars, sun damage, and wrinkles.

S-lift A modified face-lift procedure that works well on faces with only slight signs of aging.

spider veins (telangiectasias) Nonessential dilated veins that lie just beneath the surface of the skin.

subcutaneous technique A surgical procedure that tightens the skin without removing any tissue underneath it.

sublingual tranquilizer A numbing agent, placed under the tongue to dissolve prior to the operation.

superficial muscle The outermost layer of muscle that is closest to the skin.

superior palpebral fold   The upper eyelid fold.

suture   To close a wound surgically by sewing or stapling it. Also, the stitch or staple that joins together the edges of an incision.

symmetrical   The balanced and harmonious arrangement of certain aesthetic features that often help create a pleasing or attractive appearance.

tape mask   Layers of bandage that cover the entire face to promote healing after strong chemical peels.

TCA   The acronym for trichloracetic acid, which is used in skin peels.

temporal   Of or pertaining to the temples; the place where face-lift incisions and sutures are made (generally hidden within the hairline).

traumatize   To cause injury to mind or body.

tumescent liposuction   A liposuction technique that introduces dilute anesthetic solution into the skin to be treated. The fluid causes the area to balloon, ensuring minimal discomfort to the patient, making aspiration of the fat easier, and reducing postoperative discomfort.

tummy tuck (abdominoplasty)   A surgical procedure that flattens the stomach by removing fatty deposits, excess fat, and skin.

UAL (ultrasound-assisted liposuction)   A surgical technique that uses ultrasonic sound waves to break down the fat while removing it. Because UAL removes fat more discriminately, there is less blood and tissue loss and usually fewer traumas to the treated area.

ultrapulsed laser   A form of laser that delivers light in very rapid, extremely short bursts.

ultrasound   A developing technology that uses sound waves to break up fat for easier removal. See *UAL.*

undermining   Separating skin and fat from underlying tissue; once the layers are undermined, they can be excised, lifted, or redraped, as in a face lift.

varicose veins   Veins in the leg that are responsible for carrying blood back to the heart, which can become unusually enlarged or swollen by the demands of upward circulation.

w-plasty; z-plasty   Common surgical techniques used to lengthen contracted scar tissue and reorient scars so that they more closely conform to natural skin lines and creases, making them less noticeable. The letters describe the incision pattern.

Zyderm; Zyplast   Proprietary products containing collagen, used to fill out fine wrinkles. Zyderm tends to be used for lines, while Zyplast is better suited for more extreme corrections.

Resources

Products

Information on the following products can be obtained directly from the manufacturers.

SinEcch. This all-natural medicine can help reduce postsurgical bruising and swelling. Contact Alpine Pharmaceuticals at 1-888-746-3224.

SoftForm Implants. Made of ePTFE (expanded polytetrafluoroethylene), a variation of the biocompatible polymer that's used in heart transplants, tubular SoftForm allows tissue to grow inside as well as around it. For consumer information or the names of doctors trained in its use, contact Collagen Corporation at 1-800-227-8933.

The following popular products are available at stores that feature special nursing and hospital aid products:

DenTips. Antiseptic sponge swabs to clean and manage oral hygiene following surgery. Contact Medline Industries, 1200 Town Line, Mundelein, IL 60060-4486; 1-847-949-5500.

Kold kompress. Small, reusable cold compresses. Contact Physician & Nurses Manufacturing, 100 Forest Avenue, Hudson, MA; 1-978-562-7571.

Underbed Pads. Disposable pads that absorb postsurgical bleeding and oozing. Contact Griffon Medical Products, 80 Manheim Avenue, Bridgeton, NJ 08302; 1-609-455-6870.

Visual Healthware. Oversized sunglasses that cover signs of bruising and sutures following eye surgery. Contact Yorktowne Optical Co., Inc., 1720 York County Industrial Park, Emigsville, PA 17318; 1-717-767-6406.

The following postsurgical camouflage kits and make-up are available at leading department stores or by calling direct:

Clinique Advanced Concealer. Matte for easier skin matching. Call 1-212-572-3800.

Lancome's Palette Pro Complexion Perfecting Kit. A black compact with a little of each color toner. Call 1-800-LANCOME.

La Prairie's Camouflage Kit. Contains everything you need to conceal. Call 1-800-821-5718.

Linda Seidel Transforming Cosmetics. Natural cover cream with titanium dioxide for full coverage. Call 1-888-441-2424.

Stila Face Concealer. For scars and brown spots. Call 1-800-883-0400.

On the Internet

www.ahd.com   The American Hospital Directory. Provides comparative data for most hospitals, including services provided, hospital characteristics, outpatient facilities, and hospital performance.

www.aslms.org   American Society for Laser Medicine and Surgery, Inc. World's largest scientific organization dedicated to advancing medical laser applications.

www.certifieddoctor.org   Allows consumers to search for board-certified physicians by specialty and geographic area, and to verify credentials of individual physicians free of charge.

www.cosmeticscop.com   Provides information on innovative new products and unmasks the overpromise found in many overpriced beauty goods. Reams of useful information and hot tips. Findings and research are provided by the successful author of *Don't Go to the Cosmetic Counter Without Me,* Paula Begoun.

www.cosmeticsurgery.org   American Academy of Cosmetic Surgery. Provides valuable information about cosmetic procedures and help in selecting board-certified cosmetic surgeons.

www.intelihealth.com   Johns Hopkins health information. A deep index of brand names and generic names of drugs. What to know about each and questions to ask your doctor.

www.merck.com   Seventeenth edition of *Merck Manual of Diagnosis and Therapy,* available early in 1999. This site has extensive information on product news, research, and so on.

www.nih.gov   Over 3,500 medical journals with 30,000 new articles added monthly. This is a government-sponsored database, part of the National Institute of Health. Once online, use the NIH search engine; then type in the word Medline. Search by surgery type (for example, face lift) or other feature.

www.surgery.org American Society for Aesthetic Plastic Surgery, Inc. Search for board-certified plastic surgeons by geography; provides other useful information.

www.thriveonline.com Provides extensive consumer information, with broad coverage of nutrition, drugs, general health, and surgeries. Doctors will answer your questions via e-mail.

www.wlbeauty.com An independent research and consulting resource for cosmetic surgery prospects that provides facts, trends, and other useful patient information.

Organizations

Medical boards

To determine whether your surgeon is board certified for the procedure you're considering, contact one of these resources:

The American Board of Anesthesiology
4101 Lake Boone Trail
The Summit, Suite 510
Raleigh, NC 27606
1-919-881-2570

The American Board of Dermatology
Henry Ford Hospital
One Ford Place
Detroit, MI 48202-3450
1-313-874-1088

The American Board of Ophthalmology
111 Presidential Boulevard, Suite 241
Bala Cynwyd, PA 19004
1-610-664-1175

The American Board of Otolaryngology
2211 Norfolk, Suite 800
Houston, TX 77098-4044
1-713-528-6200

The American Board of Plastic Surgery
Seven Penn Center, Suite 400
Philadelphia, PA 19103-2204
1-215-587-9322

Medical and other societies

These organizations often have useful consumer information and brochures:

AAAI Physicians' Referral and Information
Line (for information on allergies, asthma, and immune therapies)
1-800-822-2762

American Academy of Cosmetic Surgery
410 North Michigan Avenue
Chicago, IL 60611-4267
1-312-527-6713
Fax: 1-312-644-1815
E-mail: *aacs@sba.com*

American Academy of Facial, Plastic, and
Reconstructive Surgery
1101 Vermont Avenue NW, Suite 404, Department MC
Washington, DC 20005
1-800-332-3223

American Association of Nurse Anesthetists
222 South Prospect Avenue
Park Ridge, IL 60068-4001
1-847-692-7050
Fax: 1-847-692-6968

American Medical Association
515 North State Street
Chicago, IL 60610
1-312-464-5000

American Society for Aesthetic Plastic
    Surgery, Inc.
444 East Algonquin Road
Arlington Heights, IL 60005
1-800-814-7148 or 1-847-228-9274
E-mail: *asapscom@surgery.org*

American Society for Laser Medicine and
    Surgery, Inc.
2404 Stewart Square
Wausau, WI 54401
1-715-845-9283
E-mail: *aslms@dwave.net*

American Society of Plastic and
    Reconstructive Surgeons, Inc.
444 East Algonquin Road
Arlington Heights, IL 60005-4664
1-800-635-0635 or 1-847-228-9000

Surgical site accreditation

The Accreditation Association for Ambulatory
    Health Care
9933 Lawler Avenue
Skokie, IL 60077
1-847-676-9610

The American Association for Accreditation
of Ambulatory Surgery Facilities
1201 Allanson Road
Mundelein, IL 60060
1-847-949-6058

The Joint Commission on Accreditation of
Healthcare Organizations
1 Renaissance Boulevard
Oakbrook Terrace, IL 60181
1-630-916-5600

Teaching hospitals

Frequently a number of top teaching hospitals offer
some cosmetic surgery procedures by residents at a
lower cost. These surgeries are performed under
the rigorous supervision of experienced, board-
certified cosmetic surgeons. As with all cosmetic
surgery, expect a thorough preoperative consultation and all necessary postoperative follow-up care.

California
Cedars of Sinai
8700 Beverly Blvd.
Los Angeles, CA 90048
1-310-855-5000

UCLA Medical Center
10833 Le Conte Avenue
Los Angeles, CA 90095
1-310-825-9111

University of CA
500 Parnassus Avenue
San Francisco, CA 94122
1-415-476-9000

Connecticut
Yale New Haven Hospital
20 York Street
New Haven, CT 06510
1-203-688-4242

District of Columbia
Georgetown University
3800 Reservoir Road NW
Washington. DC 20007
1-202-784-2000

Florida
Jackson Memorial Hospital
1611 NW 12th Street
Miami, FL 33136
1-305-585-5798

Georgia
Emory University Hospital
1364 Clifton Road
Atlanta, GA 30322
1-404-712-7021

Illinois
Rush-Presbyterian-Saint Lukes
1653 West Congress Parkway
Chicago, IL 60612
1-312-942-5000

University of Chicago
5841 South Maryland Avenue
Chicago, IL 60637
1-773-702-1000

Maryland
Johns Hopkins Hospital
600 North Wolfe Street
Baltimore, MD 21287
1-410-955-5000

Massachusetts
Boston University Hospital
720 Harrison Street
Suite 700
Boston, MA 02116
1-617-638-8000

Massachusetts General
55 Fruit Street
Boston, MA 02114
1-617-726-2000

Michigan
University of Michigan Medical Center
1500 East Medical Center Drive
Ann Arbor, MI 48109
1-313-936-4000

New York
Lenox Hill Hospital
100 East 77th Street
New York, New York 10021
1-212-434-2400

Manhattan Eye, Ear & Throat
210 East 64th Street
New York, NY 10021
1-212-838-9200

New York University Hospital
560 First Avenue
New York, NY 10016
1-212-263-5180

Ohio
Mt. Carmel Medical Center
793 West 8th Street
Columbus, OH 43222
1-614-234-5000

Ohio State University Hospital
450 West 10th Street
Columbus, OH 43210
1-614-293-5000

Tennessee
Baptist Hospital
2000 Church Street
Nashville, TN 37236
1-615-329-5555

Vanderbilt University Medical Center
Plastic Surgery Department
230 Medical Center South
Nashville, TN 37232
1-615-936-0160

Texas
Baylor University Hospital
3500 Gaston Avenue
Dallas, TX 75246
1-214-820-0111

For other hospitals, you can also check:

The American Hospital Directory
620 West Main Street
Suite 200A
Louisville, KY
1-800-577-8070
Web address: **www.ahd.com**

Experts

*Tori Kamppi, R.N., Dermatologic
Nurse/Esthetician.* Specializes in treatments
before and after cosmetic surgery. Rates vary
according to treatment. Contact: 330 East
79th Street, New York, NY 10021; 1-212-
861-3886.

Wendy Lewis & Company, Ltd. Independent,
third-party private consultant for patients
considering cosmetic surgery; recommends
prospective surgeons based on each client's
needs, then reviews consultation feedback
and prospect's reaction to surgeon. (No fees
from doctors for her referrals.) Does searches
for clients in other markets; works by e-mail,
telephone, and, locally, by private appointments, preferably in person. $100 per hour.
Contact 201 East 79th Street, New York, NY
10021; 1-212-861-6148.

Post-surgery hideaways

The Carlyle, 35 East 76th Street New York, NY
10021; 1-800-227-5737. Near major hospitals
and top surgeons' offices. The service, style,
and discretion here often attract recovering
postop plastic surgery patients. Every room
has a direct line to a nearby pharmacy.

Doubletree Grand, 1717 North Bayshore Drive,
Biscayne Bay, Miami, FL 33132; 1-305-372-
0313. Rents fully furnished condos for longer
stays, is right on the water, and is close to
Columbia Cedars Medical Center.

The Landry Tower Hotel, 411 North
Washington Avenue, Suite 5300, Dallas, TX
75246; 1-214-818-6300. Located five minutes
from downtown Dallas, this is on the same
floor as the Dallas Day Surgery Center. The
six rooms specifically reserved for plastic
surgery patients offer hospital beds and
queen-size beds for family, along with TVs
and VCRs. Nurses are stationed from early

evening to morning. The fitness center offers massages and saunas.

Le Palais Chantique at the Century Plaza Hotel (Towers), 2055 Avenue of Stars, Beverly Hills, CA 90067; 1-310-277-2270. Located within the hotel, this retreat provides one nurse for every three patients, a chauffeured car to and from postop doctor's appointments, and plenty of special attention. Nurses check on patients every 15 minutes for the first 24 hours.

Loews Vanderbilt Plaza Hotel, 2100 West End Avenue, Nashville, TN 37203; 1-800-336-3335. One block from Baptist Hospital. Rated at four stars, it has an in-house fitness center.

The Peninsula, 9882 Little Santa Monica Blvd., Beverly Hills, CA 90212; 1-800-462-7899. Patients are escorted directly to the hotel's villas for private VIP treatment.

Water's Edge Laser & Surgery Center, 210 East Osceola Street, Stuart, FL 34994; 1-800-426-8968. E-mail: *coop@watersedgesurg.com;* Web address: **www.watersedgesurg.com**. Skilled-care facility owned and operated by and for the patients of Dr. Robert N. Cooper. Nursing care is provided 24 hours a day, 365 days a year. Freshly prepared gourmet meals; phones with voice mail and 25-inch televisions in each room; temperature control; housekeeping and personal laundry service. Surgeon visits each patient twice a day.

Further Reading

Books

Atlas of the Human Body (Harper Perennial, 1994). A wonderful, simple-to-read and beautifully illustrated explanation of the human anatomy. For cosmetic surgery buffs who want to really grasp the underpinnings of their procedure by looking within the body to see which areas the surgeon will undermine, excise, or treat.

Are You Considering Cosmetic Surgery? Robin K. Levinson and Arthur William Perry (Avon, 1997). An overview of the procedures presented in a question and answer format. The book reveals a number of interesting variables in an easy-to-read format, complete with a helpful glossary. No illustrations.

Beauty and the Beam: Your Complete Guide to Cosmetic Laser Surgery, Deborah S. Sarnoff and Joan Swirsky (Quality Medical Publications, 1998). An excellent laser primer that describes leading and evolving innovative approaches to treat cosmetic (and other) skin issues.

The Beauty Bible, Paula Begoun (Beginning Press, 1997). Packed with tips about the latest in beauty products.

The Complete Guide to Cosmetic Facial Surgery, John A. McCurdy, Jr., M.D. (Lifetime Books, 1993). Remains an informative source for varied approaches to facial cosmetic surgery. Presents the dynamics of skin, tissue, and other key factors that make each person's recovery and results so individual. Amply illustrated with black-and-white photographs and drawings.

Don't Go to the Cosmetic Counter Without Me (3rd edition), Paula Begoun (Beginning Press, 1996). A guide to innovative new beauty products; unmasks the overpromise found in many overpriced beauty goods. Reams of useful information and hot tips.

The Essential Guide to Cosmetic Laser Surgery: The Revolutionary New Way to Erase Wrinkles, Age Spots, Scars, Birthmarks, Moles, Tattoos . . . And How, Tina S. Alster, et al (Alliance Publishing, 1997). Written by a highly respected, top dermatologist who explains how lasers can treat a number of skin irregularities and which laser treatment is best suited for anti-aging approaches. Emerging applications are also introduced to the reader.

Everything You Ever Wanted to Know About Cosmetic Surgery But Couldn't Afford to Ask, Alan Gaynor, M.D. (Broadway Books, 1998). An informative, sometimes amusing summary of a successful practice of a west coast physician and his state-of-the-art approach to varied methodologies.

The Face Book, American Academy of Facial Plastic and Reconstructive Surgery, Inc. (1997). A good exploratory of what common procedures can accomplish in modifying facial features. Well written and illustrated with color photographs.

Nips & Tucks: Everything You Must Know Before Having Cosmetic Surgery, Diana Barry (General Pub Group, 1996). A basic primer for women considering the more popular operations, including reconstructive breast surgery. Cost, time of operation, and postoperative expectations are described well; practically each procedure has an accompanying illustration.

Plastic Surgery: Everything You Need to Know—Before, During, and After, Richard A. Marfuggi (Perigee, 1998). Intelligent summary of many procedures, realistic expectations, and red flags to be on the look out for. Photographs used throughout and a layperson's glossary help keep you informed about procedures.

Plastic Surgery Hopscotch: A Resource Guide for Those Considering Cosmetic Surgery, Miriam Ingersoll (Editor) (Carmania Books, 1995). A good exploratory of what cosmetic surgery entails and the risks and recovery requirements that are often underplayed or minimized by cosmetic doctors. The author cites the downside potential in greater detail than most books and asks each reader to consider the most important question: Is cosmetic surgery worth the cost and risks?

Venus Envy: A History of Cosmetic Surgery, Elizabeth Haiken (Johns Hopkins University Press, 1997).

Welcome to Your Facelift: What to Expect Before, During, and After Cosmetic Surgery, Helen Bransford (Doubleday, 1997). A witty insider's look at the face-lift process from her husband's verbal slip that precipitated her quest up to the final results. This breezy yet intelligent first-person account covers it all, and also details what many books do not: day-after photos coupled with an accurate recovery progress.

What Your Doctor Can't Tell You About Cosmetic Surgery, Joyce D. Nash (New Harbinger Publications, 1995). An intelligent, well-documented survey of the field of cosmetic surgery written by a former patient who eventually loved her results but was totally unprepared for the postoperative recovery: pain, swelling, and a longer than anticipated recovery. The book is heavily researched and alerts the reader to a number of troubling oversights by doctors. With its slight academic bent, absorbing all the contents cover to cover may demand too much from the average reader.

The Youth Corridor, Gerald Imber, M.D. (William Morrow & Co., 1998). An in-depth discussion of the dynamics of the female face, how it ages, and which innovative procedures can rejuvenate one's face. Bright and intelligent descriptions by one of the country's leading surgeons who also popularized the S-lift. Drawings depict how each facial surgery is performed and where sutures are typically placed.

Newsletters

Cosmetic Connection. A make-up diva and her panel of experts give you the skinny of the world of beauty products, locates hard-to-find make-up products, and publishes a free on-line newsletter: **www.kleinman.com/cosmetics**.

Cosmetic Counter Update. The cosmetic cop blows the lid off of misleading beauty products and false advertising claims so that you can shop wisely and save at seductively expensive beauty counters. Packed with expert tips and clever information. Contact 5418 South Brandon Street, Seattle, WA 98118.

WL Beauty Watch. Up-to-the-minute news about cosmetic surgery trends, innovative procedures, postoperative products, interviews with surgeons, and industry scuttlebutt. Accepts no advertising or payments from doctors and maintains an independent point of view. Contact 201 East 79th Street, New York, NY 10021.

Magazine articles

"Bend Me, Shape Me," *New York,* July 15, 1996. What procedures (and the costs) are proposed by leading New York City cosmetic doctors to improve the appearance of a perfectly attractive, young writer who reported the story undercover.

"A Fly on the Wall at the Plastic Surgeons' Ball," *American Health,* January/February

1998. An amazing and amusing trek through a major medical conference and networking social of leading cosmetic physicians and their practically perfect spouses. Color photographs.

"A Nip Here and a Tuck There But Who Will I Be in the Morning?" *The London Times Weekend,* Saturday, April 25, 1998. What the city of London offers for appearance enhancement.

"Meeting Dr. Right," *Allure,* September 1997. A skeptical peek at the emerging world of beauty consultants and how all-too-eager prospects are shuttled (rather than independently advised) through the process.

"Ten Things Your Plastic Surgeon Won't Tell You," *Smart Money,* January 1998. A smart overview of the cosmetic surgery field and how many prospects can be taken advantage of unwittingly.

Statistics

Popularity of Procedures

When asked what procedures they would consider having done if they were to undergo facial plastic surgery, adult Americans responded:

Face Lift	23.0%
Rhinoplasty	18.0%
Skin Resurfacing	17.0%
Blepharoplasty	9.0%
Facial/Neck Liposuction	1.0%
Other	3.0%
None	15.0%
Don't Know/Refused to Answer	17.0%

(Information gathered by Wirthlin Worldwide for the American Academy of Facial Plastic and Reconstructive Surgery, July 30, 1997. Study of 1,007 adult Americans, margin of error is ±3.1 percentage points in 95 out of 100. Any variation in reported percentages of ±1% is due to rounding.)

Favorite facial feature

When asked what they considered to be their favorite facial feature, adult Americans responded:

Eyes	72.0%
Lips	7.0%
Cheeks	6.0%
Nose	5.0%
Chin	3.0%
Other	1.0%
All	1.0%
None	1.0%
Don't Know/Refused to Answer	4.0%

(Information gathered by Wirthlin Worldwide for the American Academy of Facial Plastic and Reconstructive Surgery, July 30, 1997. Study of 1,007 adult Americans, margin of error is ±3.1 percentage points in 95 out of 100. Any variation in reported percentages of ±1% is due to rounding.)

Number of procedures performed in a year (average per person)

Men	
Rhinoplasty	21.7
Hair Transplant	14.9
Filler Injections	12.8
Blepharoplasty	11.4
Chemical Peels	8.2
Face Lift	5.9
Laser Resurfacing	5.8
Facial/Neck Liposuction	5.0
Cheek/Chin Augmentation	4.7
Otoplasty	3.9
Forehead Lift	3.7

Women	
Chemical Peels	81.1
Filler Injections	48.7
Blepharoplasty	38.7
Rhinoplasty	36.7
Laser Resurfacing	35.1
Face Lift	25.5
Facial/Neck Liposuction	17.1
Forehead Lift	15.1
Cheek/Chin Augmentation	10.5
Otoplasty	4.9
Hair Transplant	1.6

(Information gathered by Wirthlin Worldwide for the American Academy of Facial Plastic and Reconstructive Surgery, August 1997. Margin of error is ±7.5% at the 90% confidence interval. Any variation in reported percentages of ±1% is due to rounding.)

Average cost per procedure

Face Lift	$5,439.00
Rhinoplasty	$5,191.90
Blepharoplasty	$3,550.10
Forehead Lift	$2,900.60
Laser Resurfacing	$2,823.60
Hair Transplant	$2,694.30
Otoplasty	$2,463.00
Cheek/Chin Augmentation	$1,752.00
Facial/Neck Liposuction	$1,535.10
Chemical Peels	$691.00
Filler Injections	$487.80

(Information gathered by Wirthlin Worldwide for the American Academy of Facial Plastic and

Reconstructive Surgery, August 1997. Margin of error is ±7.5% at the 90% confidence interval. Any variation in reported percentages of ±1% is due to rounding.)

Age groups electing to have cosmetic surgery

Less than 20 years old	8.9%
20 to 29 years old	14.1%
30 to 39 years old	18.3%
40 to 49 years old	23.9%
50 to 59 years old	24.5%
60 to 69 years old	15.2%
70 to 79 years old	7.1%
Over 79 years old	4.6%

(Information gathered by Wirthlin Worldwide for the American Academy of Facial Plastic and Reconstructive Surgery, August 1997. Margin of error is ±7.5% at the 90% confidence interval. Any variation in reported percentages of ±1% is due to rounding.)

Ethnic groups electing to have cosmetic surgery

African-American	3.2%
Asian-American	4.4%
Caucasian	83.6%
Hispanic	8.0%
Other	1.0%

(Information gathered by Wirthlin Worldwide for the American Academy of Facial Plastic and Reconstructive Surgery, August 1997. Margin of error is ±7.5% at the 90% confidence interval. Any variation in reported percentages of ±1% is due to rounding.)

Total number of procedures performed in a year (average per surgeon)

Cosmetic	
Male	49.4
Female	191.4

(Information gathered by Wirthlin Worldwide for the American Academy of Facial Plastic and Reconstructive Surgery, August 1997. Margin of error is ±7.5% at the 90% confidence interval. Any variation in reported percentages of ±1% is due to rounding.)

Location where procedures are performed

Private office	47.0%
Hospital	29.4%
Free-standing surgical center	23.7%

(Information gathered by Wirthlin Worldwide for the American Academy of Facial Plastic and Reconstructive Surgery, August 1997. Margin of error is ±7.5% at the 90% confidence interval. Any variation in reported percentages of ±1% is due to rounding.)

Documents

In order for a doctor to proceed with cosmetic treatment, you must authorize the recommended procedure. A consent form can be general or specific to the procedure you are considering. (Courtesy Wendy Lewis & Co., Ltd.)

CONSENT FORM

I hereby request, authorize, and give my consent to Dr. _____ and associates or assistants to perform upon me, _____, the following operative procedure:

_____

The nature and purpose of which is:

_____

or whatever technical procedure he may deem necessary or advisable in the diagnosis or treatment of my case.

Dr. _____ and associates or assistants have thoroughly explained the surgery that is to be performed and alternative method of treatment. I fully understand the nature and purpose of the procedure and all treatment as well as all risks and complications. Since the practice of medicine and surgery is not an exact science, I realize there is no guarantee whatsoever for my surgery.

I further give permission to have such anesthetics administered as he may deem necessary or advisable.

I also give permission for him to use any of my X-rays or photographs in medical lectures or publications.

According to _____ State Law, the following risks associated with surgery and/or anesthetics have been explained in a satisfactory manner: death, brain damage, disfiguring scars, paralysis, loss of function of body organs and the loss of function of any arm or leg.

I have read and understand the above form, completed prior to signing.

SIGNATURE _____

WITNESS _____

DATE _____

Before any cosmetic surgery, you must provide a complete medical history. Most doctors or hospitals will have you complete a form similar to this one. (Courtesy Robert N. Cooper, M.D.)

MEDICAL HISTORY

PATIENT'S NAME_____ DATE_____

AGE_____ HEIGHT_____ WEIGHT_____

DATE OF LAST PHYSICAL_____

NAME, ADDRESS AND TELEPHONE # OF DOCTOR_____

_____

DRUG ALLERGIES_____

DRUG SENSITIVITIES_____

HAVE YOU **EVER** HAD A COLD SORE ON YOUR MOUTH?_____
PREVIOUS SURGERY (PLEASE LIST)

OPERATION	YEAR	ANESTHESIA (LOCAL/GENERAL)

SERIOUS ILLNESSES OR HOSPITALIZATIONS (PLEASE LIST)

LIST ALL THE MEDICATIONS YOU ARE NOW TAKING AND THEIR DOSAGES INCLUDING OVER THE COUNTER DRUGS (I.E. ASPIRIN, VITAMINS)

COULD YOU POSSIBLY BE PREGNANT? NO_____ YES_____

NUMBER OF PREGNANCIES_____ NUMBER OF LIVE BIRTHS_____

PLEASE COMPLETE THE REVERSE SIDE OF THIS FORM

DATE OF LAST MAMMOGRAM_____

HAVE YOU EVER HAD A BLOOD TRANSFUSION? NO_____ YES_____

WHAT IS YOUR DAILY CONSUMPTION OF THE FOLLOWING?

TOBACCO _____ ALCOHOL _____

IF YOU EVER SMOKED IN THE PAST, HOW MUCH, HOW LONG AND WHEN DID

YOU STOP?_____

DO YOU USE RETIN-A?_____HOW OFTEN?_____WHAT %_____

DO YOU USE ALPHA HYDROX (GLYCOLIC)?_____HOW OFTEN?_____
MEDICAL HISTORY-CHECK IF YOU HAVE EVER HAD ANY OF THE FOLLOWING:

MALIGNANT HYPERTHERMIA	NO_____	YES_____
RADIATION THERAPY FOR ACNE AS A CHILD	NO_____	YES_____
TUBERCULOSIS	NO_____	YES_____
CANCER	NO_____	YES_____
DIABETES	NO_____	YES_____
HEART DISEASE	NO_____	YES_____
HIGH BLOOD PRESSURE	NO_____	YES_____
LUNG DISEASE	NO_____	YES_____
KIDNEY DISEASE	NO_____	YES_____
BLOOD/BLEEDING DISORDERS	NO_____	YES_____
ASTHMA	NO_____	YES_____
MENTAL ILLNESS	NO_____	YES_____
GASTROINTESTINAL	NO_____	YES_____
HEPATITIS/LIVER DISEASE	NO_____	YES_____
OTHER	_____	

Every patient is entitled to certain rights, as outlined here.
(Courtesy Wendy Lewis & Co., Ltd.)

---

1   A PATIENT'S BILL OF RIGHTS

        M.D. P.C. presents a Patient's Bill of Rights with the expectation
that observance of these rights will contribute to more effective patient care and
greater satisfaction for the patient, his physician, and the group organization. It
is recognized that a personal relationship between the physician and the patient is
essential for the provision of proper medical care. The traditional physician-patient
relationship takes on a new dimension when care is rendered within an organizational
structure. Legal precedent has established that the facility itself also has a
responsibility to the patient. It is in recognition of these factors that these
rights are affirmed.

1. The patient has the right to considerate and respectful care.

2.   The patient has the right to obtain from his physician complete current
information concerning his diagnosis, treatment and prognosis in terms the patient
can be reasonably expected to understand. When it is not medically advisable to give
such information to the patient, the information should be made available to an
appropriate person on his behalf. He has the right to know, by name, the physician
responsible for coordinating his care.

3. The patient has the right to receive from his physician information necessary to
give informed consent prior to the start of any procedure and/or treatment. Except
in emergencies, such information for informed consent should include but not
necessarily be limited to the specific procedure and/or treatment, the medically
significant risks involved, and the probable duration of incapacitation.   Where
medically significant alternatives for care or treatment exist, or when the patient
requests information concerning medical alternatives, the patient has the right to
know the name of the person responsible for the procedures and/or treatment.

4. The patient has the right to refuse treatment to the extent permitted by law and
to be informed of the medical consequences of his action.

5. The patient has the right to every consideration of his privacy concerning his own
medical care program.   discussion, consultation, examination, and treatment are
confidential and should be conducted discreetly. Those not directly involved in his
care must have the permission of the patient to be present.

6. The patient has the right to expect that all communications and records pertaining
to his care should be treated as confidential.

7. The patient has the right to expect that within its capacity,   M.D.
P.C. must provide evaluation, service, and/or referral as indicated by the urgency
of the case. When medically permissible, a patient may be transferred to another
facility only after he has received complete information and explanation concerning
the needs for and alternatives to such a transfer. The institution to which the
patient is to be transferred must first have accepted the patient for transfer.

8.   The patient has the right to obtain information as to any relationship of this
facility to other health care and educational institutions insofar as his care is
concerned.   The patient has the right to obtain information as to the existence of
any professional relationships among individuals, by name, who are treating him.

9.   The patient has the right to be advised if   M.D. P.C. proposes
to engage in or perform human experimentation affecting his care or treatment. The
patient has the right to refuse to participate in such research projects.

10. The patient has the right to expect reasonable continuity of care. He has the

right to know in advance what appointment times and physicians are available and where. The patient has the right to expect that his facility will provide a mechanism whereby he is informed by his physician or a delegate of the physician of the patient's continuing health care requirements following discharge.

11.   The patient has the right to examine and receive an explanation of his bill regardless of source of payment.

12.   The patient has the right to know what our facility rules and regulations apply to his conduct as a patient.

No catalog of rights can guarantee for the patient the kind of treatment he has a right to expect.   This facility has many functions to perform, including the prevention and treatment of disease, the education of both health professionals and patients, and the conduct of clinical research.   All these activities must be conducted with an overriding concern for the patient, and, above all, the recognition of his dignity as a human being.   Success in achieving this recognition assures success in the defense of the rights of the patient.

PATIENT RESPONSIBILITIES

It is the patient's responsibility to fully participate in decisions involving his/her own health care and to accept the consequences of these decisions if complications occur.

The patient is expected to follow up on his/her doctor's instructions, take medication when prescribed, and ask questions concerning his/her own health care the he/she feels is necessary.

You will be asked about your medical history, current medications, prior operations, and allergies in order to help determine the best anesthesia for your treatment. You may also be asked to fill out a questionnaire like this one. (Courtesy American Association of Nurse Anesthetists)

The Pre-Anesthesia Questionnaire

The pre-anesthesia questionnaire is used to help prepare you for the anesthesia process and determine the best anesthetic technique for you. You will be specifically asked about your medical history, current medications, prior operations and allergies. Additional questions may include:

Yes No

❑ ❑ Have you recently had a cold or the flu?
❑ ❑ Are you allergic to latex (rubber) products?
❑ ❑ Have you experienced chest pain?
❑ ❑ Do you have a heart condition?
❑ ❑ Do you have hypertension (high blood pressure)?
❑ ❑ Do you experience shortness of breath?
❑ ❑ Do you have asthma, bronchitis, or any other breathing problem?
❑ ❑ Do you (or did you) smoke?
  Packs/day _____ Number of years _____
  Date you quit _____
❑ ❑ Do you consume alcohol?
  Drinks/week _____
❑ ❑ Do you take or have you taken recreational drugs?
❑ ❑ Have you taken cortisone (steroids) in the last six months?
❑ ❑ Do you have diabetes?
❑ ❑ Have you had hepatitis, liver disease, or jaundice?
❑ ❑ Do you have a thyroid condition?
❑ ❑ Do you have or have you had kidney disease?
❑ ❑ Do you have ulcers or other stomach disorders?
❑ ❑ Do you have a hiatal hernia?
❑ ❑ Do you have back or neck pain?
❑ ❑ Do you have numbness, weakness, or paralysis of your extremities?
❑ ❑ Do you have any muscle or nerve disease?
❑ ❑ Do you or any of your family have sickle cell trait?
❑ ❑ Have you or any blood relatives had difficulties with anesthesia?
❑ ❑ Do you have bleeding problems?
❑ ❑ Do you have loose, chipped, false teeth, or bridgework?
❑ ❑ Do you wear contact lenses?
❑ ❑ Have you ever received a blood transfusion?
❑ ❑ (Women) Are you pregnant?
  Due date _____

A

The *Unofficial Guide*™ Reader Questionnaire

If you would like to express your opinion about cosmetic surgery or this guide, please complete this questionnaire and mail it to:

The *Unofficial Guide*™ Reader Questionnaire
Macmillan Lifestyle Group
1633 Broadway, floor 7
New York, NY 10019-6785

Gender: ___ M   ___ F

Age: ___ Under 30   ___ 31–40   ___ 41–50
___ Over 50

Education: ___ High school   ___ College
___ Graduate/Professional

What is your occupation?
_____

How did you hear about this guide?
___ Friend or relative
___ Newspaper, magazine, or Internet
___ Radio or TV
___ Recommended at bookstore
___ Recommended by librarian
___ Picked it up on my own
___ Familiar with the *Unofficial Guide*™ travel series

Did you go to the bookstore specifically for a book on cosmetic surgery?   Yes ___   No ___

Have you used any other *Unofficial Guides*™?
Yes ___   No ___

If Yes, which ones?
_____
_____
_____

What other book(s) on cosmetic surgery have you purchased?

_____

_____

_____

Was this book:
___ more helpful than other(s)
___ less helpful than other(s)

Do you think this book was worth its price?
Yes ___ No ___

Did this book cover all topics related to buying or leasing a car adequately? Yes ___ No ___

Please explain your answer:

_____

_____

_____

Were there any specific sections in this book that were of particular help to you? Yes ___ No ___

Please explain your answer:

_____

_____

_____

On a scale of 1 to 10, with 10 being the best rating, how would you rate this guide? ___

What other titles would you like to see published in the *Unofficial Guide*™ series?

_____

_____

Are *Unofficial Guides*™ readily available in your area? Yes ___ No ___

Other comments:

_____

_____

_____

_____

Get the inside scoop...with the *Unofficial Guides*™!

The Unofficial Guide to Alternative Medicine
   ISBN: 0-02-862526-9   Price: $15.95

The Unofficial Guide to Buying a Home
   ISBN: 0-02-862461-0   Price: $15.95

The Unofficial Guide to Buying or Leasing a Car
   ISBN: 0-02-862524-2   Price: $15.95

The Unofficial Guide to Child Care
   ISBN: 0-02-862457-2   Price: $15.95

The Unofficial Guide to Dieting Safely
   ISBN: 0-02-862521-8   Price: $15.95

The Unofficial Guide to Eldercare
   ISBN: 0-02-862456-4   Price: $15.95

The Unofficial Guide to Hiring Contractors
   ISBN: 0-02-862460-2   Price: $15.95

The Unofficial Guide to Investing
   ISBN: 0-02-862458-0   Price: $15.95

The Unofficial Guide to Weddings
   ISBN: 0-02-862459-9   Price: $15.95

All books in the *Unofficial Guide*™ series are available at your local bookseller, or by calling 1-800-428-5331.

About the Author

E. Bingo Wyer can tell you everything you need to know about cosmetic surgery. She has written on health and beauty for many national publications, including *The New York Times, Self, Vogue, The Chicago Tribune, Allure, New York Magazine, Avenue, Esquire, Glamour, Mademoiselle,* among others. She became interested in cosmetic surgery at five years of age when she received a Mr. Potatohead as a birthday gift.